Neuroscience:
A Medical Student's Guide

David W. Karam Md,Phd

Order this book online at www.trafford.com
or email orders@trafford.com

Most Trafford titles are also available at major online book retailers.

Printed in the United States of America.

ISBN: 978-1-4669-6521-8 (sc)
ISBN: 978-1-4669-6522-5 (e)

Trafford rev. 10/19/2012

Trafford PUBLISHING® **www.trafford.com**

North America & international
toll-free: 1 888 232 4444 (USA & Canada)
phone: 250 383 6864 • fax: 812 355 4082

CONTENTS

INTRODUCTION

All that we are, all that we know, is due in part to the nervous system. The complex conscious make up of each and every one of us is unique in who we are, but relatively similar in respect to the way the nervous system makes us that way. Incredible as it seems our ability to think, to understand our environment, respond to stimuli, love, hate, learn, walk, breath and function as an organism is based on a system of chemical reactions. These reactions are carried out by specialized tissue that is collectively called the nervous system. With such a complex and delicate system of internal communication and integration, it is easy to understand the ease with which the system can be damaged, yet the system is very resilient. There has been a large amount of data that has demonstrated the ease of disruption especially early in the development of this system due to a variety of mechanisms. As clinicians, there is concern over oxygen supply, blood supply, proper growth factors, nutritional status (both at a cellular level and as an organism), exposure to toxins (alcohol, electromagnetic radiation and other teratogens). Mechanical disruption and or disturbance are a common mechanism for the dysfunction of the system. The system is also susceptible to dysfunction more with timeframes of development especially the metabolic effects of mechanical disturbances. Sporting events are a mechanism of injury and therefore disruption for humans throughout the lifespan of those participating in such events.

It has been proposed that the dysfunction that is associated with the traumatic injury that may be involved in such participation may elicit the detrimental effects well after participation has ceased. Pathologies such as dementia, Parkinsonian syndrome and other movement disorders are the best understood. In our laboratory, we have undertaken the understanding of diffuse axonal injury in relation to blast wave propagation. In this investigation, the sporting event participation that is being investigated is American football. Repetitive heading of the soccer ball during participation in a soccer match is something that has posed a concern over the possibility of traumatic brain injury over the past few years.

CHAPTER 1

ORIENTATION TO THE CENTRAL NERVOUS SYSTEM

In order to properly understand the human nervous system, a review of the structures is necessary. An in depth understanding of the basic structural make up begins with a complete review of medical terminology. In anatomy we describe things in terms of location, function, size, orientation, direction of pull and shape. In the organization of the nervous system we are concerned with orientation and as such we can imagine a quadruped animal in orientation such as a cat. We utilize terms such as rostral, dorsal, ventral, caudal in the description of location of the tissue contained in the nervous system. Rostral refers to the position closer to the cats head while the term caudal refers to the tail of the cat. The term ventral is analogous to the belly while the term dorsal refers to the back of the animal. The other terms utilized are medial, median and lateral. Median is the understanding of the midline while medial refers to being closer to the midline. Lateral is understood to mean further from the midline. We use terms such as ipsilateral that mean we are referring to the same side of the body or contralateral meaning we are referring to the opposite side of the body. When referring to both sides we will use the term bilateral. Anterior, meaning to the front is the same as when we say ventral, likewise posterior is analogous to dorsal. We use terms such as superior or cranial to indicate a position more towards the top. In Neuroanatomy we use the term afferent to indicate something that is carrying information to another structure and conversely, we use the term efferent to indicate that the information is being carried away. We use a axiom that goes like this "DAS Dorsal—Afferent-Sensory /VEM Ventral—Efferent-Motor" that holds true in most instances.

We also discuss planes of view (Sagittal, Coronal—transverse, and Horizontal). Sagittal cuts reveal right and left portions. As in the midline reference this cut is possible to be on the midline and if such is the case, it is referred to as the midsagittal cut. Coronal cuts will reveal a anterior posterior view, while the horizontal cut will produce a top-bottom view. Confusion for many medical students comes with the manner that the coronal cut is referred to in the head versus the body. In the head if the cut is perpendicular to the axis of the forebrain it is termed Coronal and this holds true to the point of the Neuraxis where the cephalic flexure. It is important to understand the planes of the view, especially in reference to viewing radiographic studies. In radiologic studies, the coronal scans are viewed as if the patient is facing the examiner. In the axial studies, the view is as if the examiner is looking upwards through the feet. These descriptors are absolute in relation to the long axis of the spinal cord and the brain.

The human nervous system is divided into the central nervous system and the peripheral nervous system. The CNS is composed of the brain and the spinal cord. Both the brain and the spinal cord are found encased in a protective layer of bone, viscous fluid and membranes called meninges. The central nervous system is the higher cognitive aspect of the nervous system. The central nervous system is also subdivided into specific regions such as the cerebral hemispheres, the thalamus, the pons, the cerebellum the medulla, and the spinal cord. These regions will be discussed in greater detail in subsequent chapters. The brain is composed of the outer cortex, composed predominately of grey matter. Microscopic examination has shown that the grey matter is composed mainly of the cell bodies thus giving it the grayish coloration. This is contrasted by the inner white matter that is mainly the axons that will compromise the paths or the tracts of the brain. Within the inner aspects of the brain are fluid filled voids that are called ventricles. These ventricles are filled with cerebrospinal fluid and are demonstrated on radiographic studies. The size and shape of these compartments may indicate pathology.

The spinal cord on the other hand is a reversal of the brain in regards to the histologic and cytoarchitectural make up between the grey and white matter. In the spinal cord, the grey matter is located in the central aspects, while the white matter occupies the peripheral position. The spinal cord contains two enlargements, a cervical and a lumbar enlargement that will be discussed in detail later in this book. The spinal cord is a neural tube like structure that terminates in the lumbar region at the conus medullaris. Students always ask how large is the spinal cord and a general rule is that is about the size of the students 5th digit. In adults the termination is at the level of L2 in adults and L3 in a newborn. This discrepancy between these two structures is found due to the growth and development of the spinal cord versus the boney spinal column. The vertebral column grows more rapidly than the spinal cord and as such stretches the spinal cord. There are 12 cranial nerves that are seen to exit from the bony protection of the skull on the ventral surface of the brain (exception is the Trochlear nerve CN4) and 31 pairs of spinal nerves that exit the spinal cord. These cranial nerves are actually considered as part of the peripheral nervous system.

The peripheral nervous system is made up of the nerves that will connect the structures outside the CNS to the CNS. Connection to the CNS and integration is via the 31 pairs of spinal nerves, 8 cervical, 12 thoracic, 5 lumbar, 5 sacral, and a single coccygeal. The manner that the spinal nerves are formed is noteworthy as they form from the joining of a dorsal and a ventral root thus producing a spinal nerve. The dorsal root contains a ganglion that is located within the intervertebral foramen and that can have clinical implications. The motor fibers are found to posse a cell body within the central nervous system and a sensory root that will form a sensory ganglion that is considered outside the central nervous system. Structures within the CNS will have some specific terms that indicate specific tissue types and or function. Nucleus (individually) nuclei (plural) indicates that we are referring to a collection of functionally related nerve cell bodies located within the CNS. The term column indicated that we are referring to a collection of functionally related nerve cell bodies that respond to like stimuli with a like response to stimuli, in the cerebral cortex or collection of functionally related nerve cell bodies that run through a portion or the entirety of the spinal cord. A layer of tissue in neuroanatomy is termed as either a lamina, or strata (stratum) and in indicative of functionally related cells that will form a layer of tissue but that runs parallel to the plane of the larger neuronal structure associated to it. A tract in Neuroanatomy may have several names, fasciculus (fasciculi), lemniscus (lemnisci) indicates a reference to a collection of tissue that are axons and that are running parallel to each other. The term funiculus (funiculi) refers to several fasciculi running in parallel.

The peripheral nervous system is composed of the cranial nerves, the spinal nerves, and the ganglia associated to them.

CRANIAL NERVES OF THE PERIPHERAL NERVOUS SYSTEM

NUMBER	NAME	COMPONENT	FUNCTION	ORIGIN
I	Olfactory	Sensory	Smell / olfaction	Telencephelon
II	Optic	Sensory	Vision	Diencephelon
III	Occulomotor	Mixed	Eye movement	Mesencephelon
IV	Trochlear	Motor	Eye movement	Mesencephelon
V	Trigeminal	Mixed	Sensation from the Face and mouth Mastication	Metencephelon
VI	Abducens	Motor	Eye movement	Metencephelon
VII	Facial	Mixed	Facial expression Taste	Metencephelon
VIII	Vestibulocochlear	Sensory	Hearing & Balance	Metencephelon

VIV	Glossopharyngeal	Mixed	Sensation from the Pharynx, taste buds, Vascular system & Gag reflex	Myelencephelon
X	Vagus	Mixed	Autonomic control And sensation	Myelencephelon
XI	Spinal Accessory	Motor	Shoulder & Neck Movement	Myelencephelon
XII	Hypoglossal	Motor	Tongue movement	Myelencephelon

The peripheral nervous system is further subdivided into the somatic system and the autonomic system. The nerves of the peripheral nervous system innervate the smooth muscle, skeletal muscle and also cardiac muscle. Along with the muscle innervation, the PNS will innervate glandular epithelial tissue and contain a variety of sensory fibers. In the PNS the fibers are referred to as a ganglion when they are a group of nerve cell bodies found within a peripheral nerve root. In the peripheral nervous system the term nerve refers to the structure made of parallel arranged axons with the cell associated to it. These sensory fibers will enter the spinal cord via the posterior root, AKA. Dorsal root. Motor fibers of the peripheral system will exit via the anterior or the ventral root. As these nerves are in close proximity, they will join to form a mixed nerve; this structure will be called a spinal nerve.

The somatic nervous system is both a motor and sensory in function. The dorsal root mentioned above is the sensory component while the ventral root is the motor component. These specialty organizations are responsible for the dermatomes (sensory) and the myotomes (motor) areas utilized for clinical assessment.

There is another division of the human nervous system called the Autonomic Nervous System. The Autonomic Nervous System is quite different from the two previously mentioned anatomic divisions as it is not a true anatomic division. The Autonomic division is really a functional division that has components located in both the central nervous system and the peripheral nervous system. The Autonomic nervous system consists of neurons that innervate the cardiac muscle, smooth muscle and glandular epithelium. The autonomic nervous system has also been called the visceral nervous system or the vegetative nervous system, because its control is outside the conscious control. In reality, there are three further subdivisions of the ANS: the sympathetic, the parasympathetic and the enteric nervous system. The traditional view of the sympathetic nervous system is that it is the "Fight or flight" portion of the system while the parasympathetic nervous system is the "resting" aspect of the ANS, leaving the enteric nervous system to influence the digestive factors. It is important to understand that even though the three are described as a single unit along the ANS the enteric system is able to function independently of the other two. However, there is a tremendous amount of influence from the parasympathetic and the sympathetic system on digestion.

So how does this system function? What makes this complex system work? The human nervous system uses neurons as the basis for the electrochemical impulses that are used for producing the action of the system. It is very unusual in that it takes electrochemical energy and then transmits that into a movement in some instances or perpetuation of the impulses in others. In this system of communication, the human body utilizes these neurons as if they were the wiring of your home. It is imperative for the system to function most effectively if all the circuits are connected, however there are some redundant systems built in so that there can still be function even if some fail. In addition to this circuitry, the ability of the system to remodel itself or re-wire itself is something that we are just beginning to understand. This concept of remodeling makes tremendous sense as neurons are seen to die off during the lifetime of us as humans.

Since the human nervous system is so much like the electrical circuits that we make analogy to, it is easy to describe things in that manner. With over a billion connections that must be made, and the speed with which these connections must be made, the parallel manner that the nervous system is arranged in is best suited for humans to perform these vast numbers of connections and the speed with which they must be made.

This arrangement has been demonstrated experimentally to in fact be the best way to provide a mechanism for the tremendous numbers of synaptic transmissions that must take place in such a time compressed period. The cytoarchitectural design of the tracts, fasculi demonstrate the parallel arrangement that occurs even within the brain and the spinal cord itself. This tissue arrangement allows for rapid delivery of information but also a method for the redundant circuits that are seen in the human nervous system. There is however a serial component to the system. This aspect is seen in the manner that one neuron may communicate with another. It is this arrangement that allows a vast ability to manipulate the inputs and the outputs intensity, firing sequence to name a few.

Looking at the human nervous system, it can be described in terms of a simple electrical circuit, with a battery and resistor. In this traditional description, the battery is the power source that will produce the voltage for the system. In the human nervous system just as in the simple circuit, there must be a flow of the voltage through the system for the system to communicate information. The system depends on a difference in the voltage across the resistor for the voltage difference to be passed through the system and generate its effect. This voltage difference (V) that is generated across the resistor, or the neurons is the basis of the system's function. Malfunction in this will create impairment of the neuron transmitting the impulse. By convention, the system is described with the flow of the voltage difference moving from the negative pole of the battery towards the positive pole of the battery. In this description, it is a closed circuit. The circuit can be defined by Ohm's Law V=IR. Ohm's Law is represented as V= voltage difference across the resistor and is measured in volts and I= the current as it flows through the resistor and is measured in Ampers's with R= resistance within the resistor and is measured in Ohm's. In the nervous system, the resistance is influenced by the myelin sheath. In the human nervous system, the word potential is substituted for voltage difference. So there is a measurable amount of resistance that is possible to be derived as the electrons move through the closed circuit with means that there is a possible dissipation of the net flow of the electrons. In the electrical world, the wires will be insulated and in the human nervous system, we insulate with the myelin sheath as mentioned above. If there is a mathematical representation for the resistance of a system, then there must be a mathematical representation for the passage of those electrons. Conductance is the expression of the ease of the passing of the electrons. Conductance is expressed as G=I/R. In this formula, the conductance is (G) and is measured in Siemens (S) with the I representing the current flow across a resistor and is measured again in Amperes, and the R representing the resistance of the resistor and is still measured in Ohm's. In this system description, there is no net transfer of the charge through the resistor, can demonstrate a transfer of the charge when the current is passed across a capacitor. This differential is expressed as Q=CV. In this equation, Q represents the amount of charge that is stored within the capacitor and is measured in units called coulombs (C) and the capacitance is measured in units called farads (F).

CHAPTER 2

GENERAL ANATOMIC CONSIDERATIONS OF THE HUMAN NERVOUS SYSTEM

In order to better understand the human nervous system, a discussion of the anatomy with regard to position is imperative. In humans the brain demonstrates a curvature at the point of the junction of the midbrain—thalamus junction. This flexure is called the cephalic flexure. This flexure is important as it will allow for the increased area within the calvarium for additional brain matter. This flexure is what orients the forebrain into a position that is very close to being perpendicular to the long axis of the spinal cord. It points the anterior pole towards the "nose". Below this flexure, the posterior aspect of the brain surface and the spinal cord is considered to be a dorsal position. This description is consistent with the general anatomic-geographic orientation. The anterior aspect of the spinal cord and the anterior portion of the brainstem are considered as being ventral in position. These positions are altered slightly as one moves further toward the face in linear relationship. The positional differences are created by the aforementioned flexure. As one moves closer toward the face the position is considered rostral. The general anatomic terms of medial and lateral are used in relation to the orientation with the midline.

In agreement with general anatomic terms, medial will refer to a position that is closer to the midline, while lateral refers to a position that is further away from the midline.

The orientations of the planes of the nervous system are the same as in general anatomic descriptions. These planes are the Sagittal, Coronal and Transverse. The sagittal plane will divide the specimen into a right and left orientation. The Coronal plane will divide the specimen into an anterior posterior orientation. The transverse plane will divide the specimen into a superior and inferior orientation. With these planar orientations in mind, the orientations in viewing films of the nervous system will demonstrate the following positions, the axial views of a film are set in such a manner that one would be looking at the patient as if from the feet toward the head. The coronal view is taken with the orientation as if you are looking directly into the face of the patient. This has the patient's left side oriented to the examiner's right.

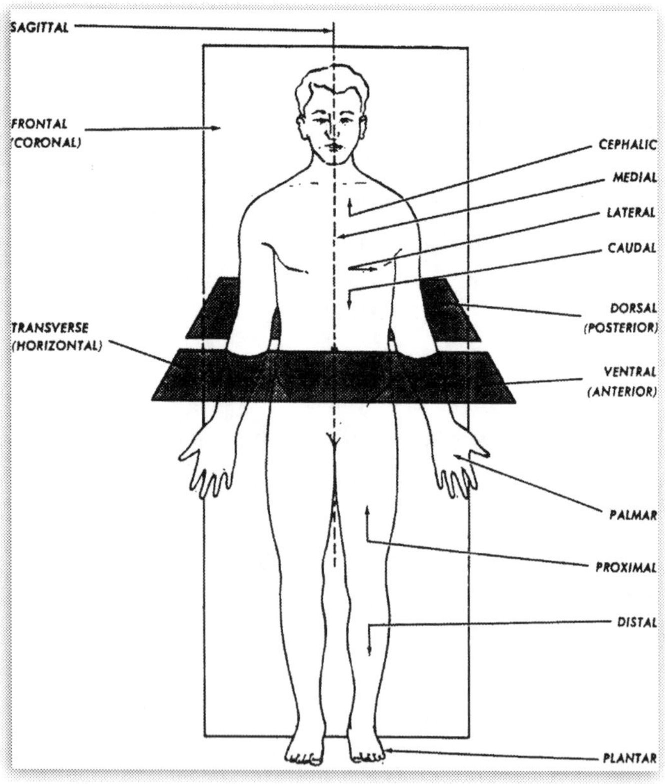

As was discussed previously in this chapter, the brain is able to be further subdivided into five specific anatomic regions. The regions are the result of the continued differentiation and proliferation of the neural tube and this development will be detailed later in chapter 5. The telencephelon, the diencephelon, the mesencephelon, the metencephelon and the myelencephelon make up the five subdivisions of the brain. The telencephelon is made of the cerebral cortex and the basal ganglia. The cerebral cortex is the most easily recognizable portion of the human brain. It consists of the surface of the brain and it is so well photographed that many of the structures are known to the student purely by photographic representation without any medical training. The elevations within this tissue mass are called gyri while the depressions are called sulci. Individual elevations are called a gyrus and the individual depressions are called a sulcus. There is a very large sulcus, the longitudinal fissure, which is seen to divide the brain into the right and left halves. These halves are then in turn designated the right and left hemispheres. Within the surface description, there are two very prominent landmarks. The central sulcus also known as the fissure of Rolando and the lateral sulcus also known as the Sylvan fissure are the most easily identifiable of the sulci. The central sulcus is seen to separate the frontal and the parietal lobes. These lobes are named for the bones of the skull that overlie them. The lateral sulcus is seen to run along the frontal and parietal lobes and is the demarcation of the temporal lobe.

The largest of the lobes of the brain is the frontal lobe. It is inclusive of the cortex rostral to the central sulcus and dorsal to the cingulated sulcus. Included in this region of the brain is the precentral gyrus. This structure houses the tissue mass that is known as the primary motor cortex. Spatially, the premotor cortex is seen to lie just rostral to the precentral gyrus. Moving more rostral, the superior, middle and the inferior frontal gyri are found. The inferior frontal gyrus is able to be further subdivided into the pars triangularis, the pars opercularis, and the pars orbitalis. These structures are of prime importance with relation to functional properties, as the pars triangularis and the pars opercularis constitute Baroca's area or the region of verbal expression. This is seen in and is indicative of the dominant hemisphere. These anatomic structures will be reviewed as a discussion of pathologic conditions is undertaken.

The parietal lobe is inclusive of the cortex that extends from the cingulate gyrus to the anterior pole of the occipital lobe. The lateral sulcus is the defining border of the parietal and the temporal lobes. The postcentral gyrus is located on the posterior aspect of the central sulcus. Within this gyrus is found the somatosensory cortex. There is also a demarcation sulcus called the intraparietal sulcus that is the demarcation line between the subdivision of the parietal lobe into the superior and inferior parietal lobules. The inferior parietal lobule is important in the interpretation of the integrative information sent via the somatosensory, auditory and visual regions of the adjacent tissue.

The temporal lobe is seen to lie within and occupy the entire middle cranial fossa. The exterior surface of the temporal lobe is subdivided into the superior, middle and inferior gyri. Anatomically, these gyri are found in a parallel orientation with the Sylvian Fissure. Within the confines of the superior aspect of the tissue, there is additional inclusive tissue that will form the auditory cortex. The duties of the primary auditory cortex are many. The primary auditory cortex is involved in the integration of the processed language center and language comprehension. Therefore, any compromise to this region of neural tissue will exhibit devastating deficit. Within the temporal lobe are the regions responsible for the processing of the visual information through the occipitotemporal and parahippocampal gyri. The primitive sense of olfaction is found to lie within a region of tissue called the uncus. The uncus is found to occupy the most medial aspect and the very tip of the parahippocampal gyrus.

Found within the most posteriocaudal aspect of the parietal and the temporal lobe is the occipital lobe. The calcarine sulcus is the large fissure that is found oriented along the medial aspect of the lobe. This is the primary visual interpretation area. The architecture of this lobe is such that the functional capacity of the lobe is oriented from a caudal to rostral manner. These are the demarcated areas of the cerebral cortex. There are continued functional divisions that are not as well anatomically defined as those mentioned previously. In these areas, the term has been used calling the tissue "synthetic lobes" due to the lack of anatomic demarcation. These synthetic lobe areas are the limbic lobe, located as a composite of tissue from the medial aspects of the frontal, temporal and the parietal lobes, and the insula that is found along the innermost aspects of the lateral sulcus. The insula is covered by the opercular cortex. Functionally, the insula is responsible for the gustatory information processing mainly. There is additional evidence as to the role of the insula in the maintenance of the cardiovascular, pulmonary and gastric functional activities. The limbic lobe on the other hand is a very complex region of tissue. The limbic lobe is functionally responsible for the expression of emotion. The limbic lobe is itself a conglomeration of tissue that is derived from the subcallosal, cingulate and the parahippocampal gyri and inclusive of the hippocampal tissue itself. The anatomic arrangement of these tissues is rather unusual in that they form a blanket of tissue surrounding the diencephelon.

Included in this mass of tissue called the cerebral cortex is the basal ganglia. The basal ganglia are made from several different regions of brain tissue within the telencephelon. These tissues consist of the caudate nucleus, the globus pallidus, the putamen, and the amygdyla. There are variations of description of these structures by grouping. If one is talking of the globus pallidus and the putamen alone, then the term used is the lenticular nucleus. If one is discussing the caudate nucleus, the putamen and the globus pallidus as a group then the term used is the corpus striatum. As the internal capsule is a band of tissue that separates the caudate and the putamen, this is not always true in functional representation as they are collectively referred to as the neostriatum.

The diencephelon is a collection of other tissue as well. It is made up of the thalamus, the hypothalamus, the subthalamus and the epithalamus. There is a unique geographic configuration to the diencephelon as well. The dorsal border of the diencephelon is generally not visible as it is overlaid with the corpus callosum and the cerebral cortex. The ventral aspect of the diencephelon is however exposed to visualization along the base of the brain. The diencephelon is composed of subdivisions of tissue as mentioned previously, and one of these subdivisions is the thalamus.

The thalamus is a very important structure within the brain. It is the main relay station for the information processing for the sensory system as the signal is being transposed to the neocortex. The thalamus is also a relay for the motor refinement pathways from the cerebellum and the primary motor cortex. There is also evidence of the thalamus and its role in the brain's regulation of sleep, arousal and its state of consciousness.

The hypothalamus is the most unique of all in its functional role within the brain. The hypothalamus is involved in such variable activities as the vegetative, cognitive functions, food intake, thirst, sleep, endocrine regulation, reproduction, thermoregulation and the post partum maternal behaviors. These incredibly wide spectrum functional implications are a clear demonstration of how any compromise of the hypothalamus can have broad spectrum and devastating consequences. Anatomically, the hypothalamus is defined by the borders of the walls and the floor of the third ventricle. The internal capsule defines the lateral border of the hypothalamus in conjunction with the subthalamic nuclei and the lenticular fasciculus. The epithalamus is the tissue that is inclusive of the pineal gland and the habenular nuclei. The role of the epithalamus is in the regulation and the integration of the diurnal rhythm. This is a small portion of the thalamic tissue. The subthalamus is seen to occupy the space inferior to the internal capsule.

The brain stem is a compilation of neural structures just as is the cortex. The brain stem is composed of the midbrain or the mesencephelon, the pons or the metencephelon, and the medulla or the myelencephelon. These structures are vastly important in their roles that include sensory, motor and vegetative roles. The motor activity of the brainstem includes the musculature of the intraoral cavity, face, head and the eyes. There is an anatomic dividing structure that will create a dorsal and ventral division. The ventral region is called the tegmentum. The dorsal region is called the tectum. The sensory inputs to the brainstem will integrate the somatosensory information from the periphery, auditory inputs from the ear, taste information and the vestibular inputs. The input is directed from the cranial nerves associated to the sense. The tegmentum is responsible for the reticular formation and the passage of a variety of ascending and descending tracts.

The mesencephelon is the smallest of the regions of the brainstem. It is also known as the midbrain. Geographically, the borders of the mesencephelon are the pineal gland with the posterior commissure and the habenular with the crus cerebri acting as the demarcation between the midbrain and the diencephelon. There is a rostral demarcation that is identified by the position of the third ventricle and the cerebral aqueduct. In the dorsal region also known as the tectum, there are two elevations of note. These are the inferior and superior colliculi. There is a bit of anatomic trivia in the only cranial nerve to exit from the dorsal aspect of the brainstem. Opposing the dorsal region in the ventral aspect is the substantia nigra and the crus cerebri.

The metencephelon or the pons is like the previously mentioned aspects, made up of several components. The ventral aspect of the pons exhibits a bulge that is identified as the pontine nuclei. These pontine nuclei are important structures in the functional capability of the brain. These fibers will provide the conduit between the cerebral cortex and the cerebellum. There are efferent projections that will emanate from the pontine nuclei that will then terminate as the middle cerebellar peduncle, the largest of the afferent pathways that lead into the cerebellum. On the dorsal surface of the pons will be the floor of the fourth ventricle. Within this ventricle are the facial colliculi. The facial colliculi is composed of the combined fibers of the facial nerve and the abducens nucleus. This surface is easily identified with visual inspection by the number of cranial nerves that are found to exit this region of the dorsal surface of the brain. The trigeminal nerve CN V has the motor and sensory roots that are seen to exit from this region. The Abducens nerve CN VI is also seen to exit in this region. The facial nerve CN VII has fibers that project form this region as well. These fibers are the motor and the intermediate nerve roots that are seen to exit from here. The vestibulocochlear nerve CN VIII, is the last remaining cranial nerve known to exit from this region.

The cerebellum is visually one of the most recognizable parts of the human brain. The cerebellum takes up the bulk of the posterior fossa of the calvarium. It receives projections from most every major sensory fiber are seen to make their way to the cerebellum. Through these inputs the cerebellum is able to interpret data regarding balance, muscle tone and fine motor control. This regulation is accomplished through negative feedback systems in place. The anatomic divisions of the cerebellum are much like that of the cortex, having a cortical and subcortical region. The dorsum of the cerebellum is separated from the occipital lobe through a very tough fibrous dural component that is called the tentorium. Tethering the cerebellum to the brainstem are the superior, middle and the inferior cerebellar peduncles. The cortex of the cerebellum is divided into two halves by the thickened band of tissue called the vermis. Each hemisphere is again subdivided, just as in the cerebral cortex. In the cerebellar hemispheres there are three lobes identified, the most rostral being the paleocerebellum with the most caudal lobe being the archicerebellum and sandwiched between the two is the paleocerebellum. Visual inspection of the cerebellum will elicit a deep sulcus that is called the primary fissure. This fissure is of importance as a landmark in identifying the demarcation of the paleocerebellum from the neocerebellum.

The medulla or the myelencephelon is the portion of the system that joins the spinal cord to the brain. It is bordered by the spinal cord caudally and running up to the caudal aspect of the pons. Identification of the adjoining point of the medulla to the spinal cord is easily made as the pyramidal decussation is seen at that point. The pyramidal tracts are seen to cover significant bulges that are the underlying inferior olivary nuclei. On the dorsal aspect of the medulla, but recessed within it will be the fourth ventricle. Inspection of the dorsal surface will yield a variety of structures from exiting cranial nerves to the tubercle Gracilis and just rostrolateral is the nucleus cuneatus. Additionally there is the tubercle formed by the underlying trigeminal tract that is known as the tuberculum cinereum. The cranial nerves that are seen to exit from the dorsal surface are the glossopharyngeal nerve CN IX; the vagas nerve CN X, the spinal accessory nerve CN XI, and the hypoglossal nerve CNXII.

CRANIAL NERVES

NUMBER	NAME	COMPONENT	FUNCTION	ORIGIN
I	Olfactory	Sensory	Smell / olfaction	Telencephelon
II	Optic	Sensory	Vision	Diencephelon
III	Occulomotor	Mixed	Eye movement	Mesencephelon
IV	Trochlear	Motor	Eye movement	Mesencephelon
V	Trigeminal	Mixed	Sensation from the Face and mouth Mastication	Metencephelon
VI	Abducens	Motor	Eye movement	Metencephelon
VII	Facial	Mixed	Facial expression Taste	Metencephelon
VIII	Vestibulocochlear	Sensory	Hearing & Balance	Metencephelon
VIV	Glossopharyngeal	Mixed	Sensation from the Pharynx, taste buds, Vascular system & Gag reflex	Myelencephelon
X	Vagus	Mixed	Autonomic control And sensation	Myelencephelon
XI	Spinal Accessory	Motor	Shoulder & Neck Movement	Myelencephelon
XII	Hypoglossal	Motor	Tongue movement	Myelencephelon

The nervous system is made up of neurons and glial cells. The basic functional unit of the nervous system is the neuron. Neurons are specialized to receive input, transmit the input as an electrical impulse, and to influence adjacent neurons or effector tissue. Neurons consist of a cell body or perikaryon or soma. There are processes that will project from the cell body; these projections are called the axon and the dendrite. As a group the neuron cell bodies are called the grey matter. Clusters of the cell bodies are functionally named as nuclei. Singular cell bodies are called nucleus. The dendrite is the process that will carry the impulse to the cell body while the axon is a singular process that will carry the impulses away from the cell body. The CNS white matter consists of bundles of axons wrapped in a protective and insulative sheath called myelin. Myelin is made of lipoproteins. The axon will terminate at a special structure called a synapse. Synapses consist of a presynaptic portion that is part of the axon itself and a space between the presynaptic terminal and the postsynaptic terminal called a synaptic cleft. The postsynaptic region is located on the effector or another neuron. The presynaptic and postsynaptic regions communicate via a release of a chemical substance called a neurotransmitter. The neurotransmitter is released within the presynaptic region due to an electrical impulse termed an action potential that will modulate its release. The neurotransmitter will be released from the presynaptic neuron from synaptic vesicles that will fuse with the presynaptic membrane to allow its release. The transmitter will diffuse across the synaptic cleft to be bound to the postsynaptic receptor. The residual neurotransmitter that is remaining in the synaptic cleft will be inactivated by a chemical reaction with AChE. This transmission of neuromodulator is unidirectional from presynaptic to postsynaptic. This transmitter may be excitatory or inhibitory depending on the neurotransmitter's chemical composition. For simplicity, the diagramming of a neural circuit has, by convention, been designated as the dendrites and the cell body will be represented by a large dot. The axon will be represented by a line with the termination being an inverted arrow at the synapse.

The nervous system functions via neurons interacting with each other. The most simplistic neural circuit is the "monosynaptic reflex arc". This type of reflex includes two neurons and only one synapse, thus the name monosynaptic. In this example of a neural circuit, the impulse or action potential is brought to the spinal cord via the dorsal root where it will exert its effect on a motor neuron. The axon of the motor neuron will transmit the action potential from the spinal cord to the skeletal muscle, which will respond by a contraction. A detailed discussion of the mechanism of action for the action potential and the mechanism of propagation of the action potential will follow in subsequent parts of this paper.

CHAPTER 3

THE CELL BIOLOGY OF NEURONS AND GLIA

There is an estimated 100 billion cells in the human adult central nervous system. The predominant cell types are glial cells and neurons. What sets nerve cells apart from other cell types is the ability to manipulate the information presented to them. It has been well published that all cells are capable of stimulus-response activity in relation to the alteration in the external environment. Neurons are able to take these general characteristics and expand upon them. This manipulation is the transformation of electrochemical energy into biochemical energy, and then back into electrochemical energy. Once this process is begun, the system has the ability to amplify the signal, temper the signal, or modify it via negative feedback. The nerve cell, in conjunction with other nerve cells is even able to perform the functions of divergence and convergence. The neuron is also capable of utilizing a variety of substances for communication, neurotransmitters or neuropeptides or neurohormones. This ability to modulate the system is due to the electrical circuit like design. By the parallel arrangement of the nerve bundles coupled with the ability to prevent degradation of the signal and use of properties of convergence and divergence, the system can modulate itself. In order to perform the function assigned a nerve cell as described above, they require vast amounts of energy in the form of glucose and oxygen. Their energy demands are so great because the function of a nerve cell entails the movement of ions across an energy gradient. The neuron is responsible for the manufacturing of the cytoskeletal components to sustain itself and the components of the cell membrane that add to the neuron's great metabolic demand. Along with sustaining its metabolic demands, the nerve cell will receive information from the periphery or from other nerves for potentiation or propagation or initiation. It must then integrate this input, and then once integrated; it must send information to either another nerve or to an effector, cell or organ.

Neurons have been shown to possess variable sizes and shapes. The most graphic demonstration of this is between the very small cerebellar cortical cell when compared to the very large Purkinje cell. Neurons have also been demonstrated to be of variable lengths, ranging from only a few micrometers to several feet. Sensory neurons are by general rule smaller than the motor neuron. Neurons do not divide again once they achieve maturity, or final differentiation. Therefore, once the cell dies, it is a permanent loss of that neuron. There is new evidence on the use of nerve growth factors and use of stem cells with neuroprogenitor cells that seem to show efficacy in replacing these neurons once that they are lost. It is not a repair but a growth of new neurons. This is very promising for neurodegenerative disorders, brain injury, diffuse axonal injury, and spinal cord injuries.

The cells of the human nervous system are generally classified as one of two major types, either neurons or the supportive cell. The neuron is the cell type known to carry the electrical signal, or action potential, while the glial cell is the major supportive cell. Glial cells will provide the nutrients required by the neuron by moving the nutrients from the blood to the cells and then removing the metabolic waste. The most important early function of a glia cell is to provide a structural lattice for the neuron to follow and thus provide a map for the neuron to insure it arrives at the correct destination. Neurons demonstrate four characteristics, they have a cell body (or perikaryon or soma), a dendrite, an axon, and terminal regions. This translates into the neuron being able to receive information, process the information, and send the information along the pathway. Neurons are further classified by the shape that they will assume, pseudounipolar, unipolar and multipolar. A neuron's cell body or soma, also called perikaryon is completely surrounded by a plasma membrane. This plasma membrane is called the neurolemma. The cell body is the metabolic and genetic control center of the neuron. This property is the same regardless of the neuron type. The cell body or perikaryon is small compared to the remainder of the neuron as measured by volume, but is extremely metabolically active. Within the cell body are the majority of the subcellular organelles. These organelles include a single large nucleolus, extensive endoplasmic reticulum (ER), golgi apparatus, ribosomes and mitochondria.

Neurons are a very complex cell type. The function that they are required to perform on a daily basis is extraordinary. In order to maintain this functional and structural job requirement the cell must provide all of its own construction materials and then must be able to transport them. In addition to the manufacturing of the building materials, the neuron must also manufacture the substances that it releases to propagate the action potential and the packaging for those substances. In the performance of these activities, the cell this eukaryotic cell will utilize the basic cellular organelles to achieve this end goal. The neuron is encased within a membrane that is called the neurolemma. It is analogous to the plasma membrane. The nucleus is the control center of the neuron just as in other eukaryotic cells. It regulates the expression of the genetic scheme of the neuron and thus dictates the behavior of the neuron. The nucleus is sequestered from the remainder of the cell cytoplasm by the nuclear membrane a double layered membrane also known as the nuclear envelope. This nuclear membrane contains openings that allow for the passage of materials in and out of the nucleus called nuclear pores. The nucleolus is the site of ribosomal RNA synthesis. In neurons these nucleoli are very prominent, owing to the increased activity required from them to meet the extreme demands for new protein synthesis. The Endoplasmic reticulum is as in other cells made up of the ribosomal studded area and the smooth area. The prototypic description of the rough endoplasmic reticulum is that it is studded with ribosomes. The endoplasmic reticulum is responsible for protein synthesis. Owing to the tremendous amount of protein synthesis required for a neuron to function, there is a very extensive endoplasmic reticulum. This extensive system of ribosomes is also the reason for the basic staining that is noted and termed as a Nissel stain. The initial portion of the tube that is designated as the endoplasmic reticulum is known as the rough endoplasmic reticulum or the RER and it is responsible for the recognition of the signal recognition particle that binds to the peptide chain and indicate that it is going to be passed to a secretory vessicle for transport based on the signal sequence. The remainder of the endoplasmic reticulum is devoid of the ribosomes and thus designated as the smooth endoplasmic reticulum (SER). The SER is responsible for the synthesis of the phospholipids. The smooth endoplasmic reticulum is also the storage unit of cellular calcium for the neuron. There will be a detailed discussion of the processes of the endoplasmic reticulum and the N-linked glycosylation that occurs within will be presented in chapter 8. The Golgi complex, AKA the Golgi apparatus is the organelle that is responsible for the O-linked glycosylation of the proteins that have been sent for modification. The golgi has two faces of note, the cis- and the trans face. Lysosomes are organelles that are responsible for the removal of the byproducts of the cell. They degrade the unused or old receptors and ligands as well as the secretory vessicles that are not reused. Lysosomes are also responsible for the degrading of the other organelles such as the mitochondria, and the endoplasmic reticulum. The lysosome maintains via an ATPase dependent proton pump a pH of approximately 5. From the lysosomes, the proteins can be sent to the endosome or the late endosomes.

The cytoskeletal proteins will be the determining factor of the neuron form. These cytoskeletal components include the neurofilaments, microfilaments and microtubules and cytoskeletal associated proteins. Projecting out from the soma is the dendrite tree and the axon. It is this structural property that is the defining point of the subcatagorization of neurons, as unipolar, multipolar, or bipolar. In the multipolar neurons, there are many dentritic endings with a lone axon. This multiple dendritic arborization produces a polygonal shaped cell. This is contrasted to the pseudounipolar /unipolar neuron that has a round shape with single projections. The position of the nucleus is of prime importance in the identification of this type of neuron as it is centrally located. Projecting from the perikaryon will be a divided branch that will become a peripheral branch and a central branch. The central branch will carry the information on to the CNS while the peripheral branch will provide sensory input to the neuron. This is very unique in that the projection serves as both the axon and the dendrite. This type of neuron is found mainly within the sensory ganglia of spinal and cranial nerves. The final subtype is the bipolar neuron. The bipolar neuron exhibits a ovoid shaped cell body. On each pole of the cell body will be the projections for the axon and the dendrite. This subtype is mainly found in sensory ganglia.

The axon emanates from the cell body at a very specific anatomic landmark, the hillock of the axon. Axons are also known in the literature as a neurite. Just as the cell body or soma or perikaryon is surrounded by a cell membrane, the axon is surrounded by a membrane called the axolemma. The cytoplasm of the axon is called the axoplasm. This axonal projection is referred to as the synaptic terminal, the terminal zone arborization or event the telodendrion. Found within the axoplasm will be large quantities of mictotubules and neurofilaments that will play a role in the movement of materials along the axon and provision of materials for the cytoarchitectural framework. This is a very important feature of an axon as they are able to travel extensive distances prior to branching. The proteins that are associated with the microtubules are designated as MAP's (microtubule associated proteins). In order for the axon to provide the materials required for the function assigned it, the axon must deliver the necessary structural and nutritional elements. In order for this to occur, the axon moves these elements by axoplasmic transport. This axoplasmic transport is done in a variable speed manner; there is fast axoplasmic transport in an anterograde or orthograde direction and fast axoplasmic transport in a retrograde direction. The fastest anterograde transport runs at a rate of 200-400mm/day and is responsible for the transport of vesicles/ neurotransmitters/ membrane proteins and lipids. Medium speed transport runs at a rate of 50-100mm/day and is responsible for the transport of mitochondria. The slow transport rate is subdivided into 2 categories a & b. The slow "a" runs at a rate of 0.2-0.1 mm/day and is responsible for the transport of protein subunits of the neurofilaments and microtubules. The slow "b" transport runs at a rate of 2-8 mm/day and is responsible for the transport of clathrin and calmodulin. The movement in this direction is accomplished through the protein kinesin. The movement of substances from the axonal terminal to the cell body is the retrograde transport mentioned above and it is directed by the protein, dynein. This mechanism of transport is in response to molecules that are ingested, such as growth factors that will require a response from the soma.

The axon carries impulses as action potentials from the point of action potential initiation, the initial segment, to the terminal bouttons or synaptic terminals. The axon within the central nervous system will terminate in very fine branched networks called terminal arbors. However, in some axons, the outpouchings or enlargements called bouttons and are found along the length of the axon and as such are called bouttons en passant. Some axons will display a swelling, smaller than the bouttons and these are called varicosities. These varicosities are also a point of signal or information transmission. This axonal projection is referred to as the synaptic terminal, the terminal zone arborization or event the telodendrion. It is this property of the excitability of the membrane that makes the axon an important part of the human nervous system. The physical characteristic of the membrane makes this excitability continue the flow of the action potential that was generated at the initial segment of the axonal hillock. The projection of the axon is a singular projection as it emerges from the perikaryon, in contrast to the dendrite. Histologically, the initial segment is important as it is devoid of the Nissel substance and thus devoid of ribosomes as described above. Axons as a whole are generally without ribosomes. This lack of ribosomes is a clear indication that the axon in not involved in the active synthesis of proteins. Axons are also known to display recurrent branches that originate at or near the soma, while other recurrent axons are seen throughout the axon.

Dendrites or dendritic trees arise from the cell body. Many are extensively arborized so that they give the appearance of a tree or bush. The collective of dendrites and their respective branches will be called the dentritic tree. The function of a dendrite is simple; receive signals from other neurons or from the peripheral receptors. If the reception is from another neuron then it is from the interneuron or the motor neuron, whereas if the connection is from the environment it is a sensory dendrite. Along the distal aspect of a dendrite are small projections called dendritic spines. It is here at the dendritic spines that the actual synaptic contact is made. This entire representation of the input portion of the dendrite is called the dendritic zone. The dendrite will become larger and thicker closer to the cell body. The dendrite is now collectively known as a primary dendrite, complete with some of the same organelles found within the cell body. It is important to note that the smaller dendrites are without organelles. However, these smaller dendrites do possess cytoskeletal elements. The larger the dendrite, the more apparent the cytoskeletal structures become. Microtubules and neurofilaments are visible as well as a variety of organelles, mitochondria, endoplasmic reticulum, polyribosomes and free ribosomes are possible to see in these larger dendrites. Neuron classification is also based upon the relationship between the axon and the dendrite in terms of length. If the axon of a multipolar neuron is extending beyond that of the dendrite it will be called a Golgi Type1. The Golgi Type 2 multipolar neuron has an axon that is no longer than that of the dendrite.

The cell body or the soma or the perikaryon is the metabolic center of the nerve. There are many mitochondria within the cell body. It is the site for the manufacturing of the macromolecules that are required for the proper functioning of a neuron. The neuron uses proteins for the majority of its processing of compounds into the macromolecules described. In the neuron, the genetic encoding of the information that is required for the formation of the proper proteins is via the DNA manufactured within the nucleus of the cell body. This genetic direction is transcribed into the RNA with further translation into the proteins utilized throughout the neuron. Because of the amount of protein required for this functional role of the neuron, there is a very extensive role for the mitochondria. The mitochondria and enzymes within the neuron provide the mechanism for this required biosynthesis of the macromolecules and the intermediary metabolism required for the generation of energy from the major biochemical pathways that produce the energy requirements. These pathways will generate the ATP via oxidative phosphorylation in the termination of the pathways. This need for so many mitochondria is evident from the reflection of the great energy requirements of the nerve. The nerve cell body will show evidence of a large nucleus and a prominent nucleolus with the requirements for the tremendous amounts of translation of the genetic information as mentioned before. Within the cytoplasm of the soma there are a great many ribosomes with a very extensive rough endoplasmic reticulum. An extensive Golgi network is also noted. Because of the extensive ribosomal content the soma will stain basophilic due to the high RNA content of the ribosomes attached to the ER. This is clinically important in diagnosis of certain metabolic disorders. The synthesis of the proteins discussed is very energy expensive. The energy requirement of a neuron is not something that is a consideration for most medical students. The rate of the synthesis of the cytosolic proteins is limited by the rate of initiation of the protein manufacturing. The production of these important cytosolic proteins has been divided into phases of initiation, elongation and finally termination. Remember that the synthesis of the cytosolic proteins must take place on the 80s subunit that will dissociate into the 40S and the 60S subunits. This entire process is extensively discussed later in this text.

CHAPTER 4

NEURON CLASSIFICATIONS

Neurons are classified into three types on the basis of cell body shape and the pattern of the emergence of the axon and dendrite. The three classifications are: multipolar, pseudounipolar, and bipolar neurons. Multipolar neurons are seen with many dendrites emerging from the cell body to give it a polygonal shape. This cell type has a single axon that will emerge from the cell body. There are many different types of multipolar neurons in the CNS. Pseudounipolar or even unipolar neurons are similar to the multipolar neurons in structure, which is they have a soma, a dendritic tree and an axon. The pseudounipolar neuron however has a centrally located cell body and only a single process. This single process of the pseudounipolar neuron has two separate parts that will bifurcate from an area close to the cell body. One process is charged with the task of carrying sensory information from the periphery, and it is thus called the peripheral branch. The other process is called the central branch, and it has a task of sending the information on to the target within the CNS. The unique feature of a pseudounipolar neuron is that the process act in conjunction with one another as a combined axon and dendrite. The more distal aspects of the peripheral process has the dendritic spines and gathers the sensory information to be sent along to the soma for integration and the central process is then responsible for the continued passage of the sensory information to the brain or spinal cord. The pseudounipolar neurons are located in a rather unique position within the nervous system, they are primarily found in the sensory ganglia of cranial nerves or spinal nerves.

Bipolar neurons are the third classification of neurons to be discussed. Bipolar neurons have a round or oval shape soma from which extends a single relatively large process. The bipolar neurons have but one process, extending from each pole of the soma. Bipolar neurons carry out a very specific function; they are used for the transmission of special senses. The function of the bipolar neurons will vary according to the location. In the olfactory system, the bipolar neurons themselves are the receptor, while in the retina; they are interspersed among the receptor cells. In contrast, bipolar neurons are the output cells in the vestibular and auditory system.

The axon is a projection that arises from the soma of a neuron. The actual point of projection is called the axonal hillock. This is a small elevation adjacent to the cell body. As the axon projects form the cell body there is a structure called the initial segment that is actually part of the axon. The initial segment is where the membrane permeability is greatest. Axonal cytoplasm, called axoplasm, contains microtubules and neurofilaments. These proteins are the structural components of the axon. These proteins are also responsible for the transport of metabolites and organelles along the length of the entire axon. Unlike dendrites, axons do not contain ribosomes. And axons may also extend for great distances. Axons within the CNS contain terminal arbors, which are fine branches at the endings of the axon. This axon terminal is then capped with a special structure, called the terminal bouton. It is this structure that is the functional aspect of the synapse between cells. In a small percentage of axons, the terminal boutons are located along the entire length of the axon. In this scenario, they are called boutons en passant. In still other axons, there are varicosities that act like boutons. These small swellings are not true boutons but they do provide a place for cell to cell communication.

In order for the neurons to continue to function, they require a constant stream of nutrients. For this to happen, the axon must provide its own nutrients. This is accomplished by axonal transport. Axonal transport is responsible for the transport of organelles ands macromolecules from the soma to the terminal bouton. This transport occurs in both directions, as the byproducts of the cellular metabolism must be transported back to the cell body for disposal. Transport from the cell body to the axonal terminal is called anterograde transport or orthograde transport. Transport in the reverse direction, from the terminal to the cell body is called retrograde transport. Anterograde transport has four variations on the manner in which organelles and nutrients are transported. There is a fast, medium and two slow components. In fast anterograde transport, the main substance transported is macromolecules containing proteins and mitochondria and some neurotransmitters. The rate of transport is 100-400 mm/day. The mechanism of this mode of transport is the protein, kinesin. The kinesin acts much like a chain of hands passing the protein vesicle from one pair to the next. The Kinesin is an ATPase molecule that requires oxidative metabolism for its function. Medium anterograde transport occurs at a rate of 50-100 mm/day. Kinesin is again the protein involved in the medium transport. A protein called dyenin brings about slow anterograde transport. Slow anterograde transport is broken down into two subtypes, a and b. Dyenin is responsible for the transport of structural proteins like actin, myosin and tubulin. This is the slow—a subtype and the rate of transport is 0.2-1.0 mm/day. The slow—b subtype is responsible for the transport of things like Clathrin, calmodulin, and other metabolic enzymes. The rate of transport in this subtype is 2-8 mm/day.

Retrograde axonal transport is of a fast nature, 50-250 mm/day. In this mode of transport, pinocytotic vesicles are re-uptaken and transported back to the soma. This mode of transport is also responsible for the return of growth factors from the terminals to the soma. The protein responsible for this transport is dyenin. The problem is that there are pathogenic problems associated with this type of transport. The rabies virus is one example of how a neurologic disease is transmitted via retrograde transport. There are many other viruses transported via retrograde transport but researchers utilize this same transport mode as a tool to investigate disease processes.

Most structures within the nervous system are formed form a related group of cell bodies. Within the CNS, clusters of functionally related nerve cell bodies are called a nucleus. If the cell bodies form a layer of cells, the term is then layer or lamina or a stratum. If these cell bodies are arranged in a columnar array, the cells are then called a column. In the cerebral cortex, this term is used for a group of cells that are related by function and by the location of the stimulus. In the spinal cord, the term refers to a longitudinal group of functionally related cells that extends for a portion, or for the entire length of the cord. In the CNS, a bundle of axons are called tracts or fasciculus or lemnisci. A group of functionally related tracts are then called a funiculus or a system. A collection of cell bodies located in the peripheral nervous system has different nomenclature. Cell bodies in the PNS are called a ganglion. In the PNS these ganglion may exhibit motor or sensory properties. The PNS has different terms for axons as well. In the PNS an axon is a nerve, a rami or a root. Neurons are also classified according to functional properties. If the neuron carries signals from the periphery to the CNS, it is called an afferent. If the neuron is designated as efferent, then its function is to carry impulses from the CNS to the effector. If the neuron has a long axon that functions in transmitting signals to a distant target or effector then they are called projection neurons. If the neuron is termed an interneuron or a local circuit cell, then it has an action of local effect. Neurons are also classified according to the neurotransmitter they utilize. If the cell contains a neurotransmitter dopamine, then it is called dopaminergic. Likewise if the neuron utilizes glutamate as its transmitter, it will be called glutaminergic.

NAME	DESCRIPTION AND EXAMPLES

CNS STRUCTURES

Nucleus—group of functionally related nerve cell bodied in the CNS.
i.e. inferior olivary nucleus, nucleus ambiguus, caudate nucleus.

Column—Group of nerve cell bodies with functional and positional Relation. Orientation is perpendicular to the plane of the cortex.
i.e. ocular dominance, columns of the visual cortex.
In the spinal cord, related nerve cell bodies that run longitudinally
Through all or part of the length of the spinal cord i.e. Clarke's columns.

Layer, Lamina, stratum—group of functionally related cells that form a layer
Parallel to the plane of the larger neural structure that includes it.
i.e. Layer IV of the cerebral cortex.

Tract, fasciculus, lemniscus—Bundle of parallel axons in the CNS.
i.e. Optic tract, Corticospinal tract, medial longitudinal fasciculus.

Funiculus—group of several parallel tracts or fasciculi.
i.e. Anterior, posterior, lateral funiculi of the spinal cord.

PNS STRUCTURES

Ganglion—group of nerve cell bodies located in peripheral nerve or a root.
Forms a visible knot.
i.e. Dorsal root ganglia, Trigeminal ganglion

Nerve, ramus, root—Peripheral structure consisting of parallel axons plus the Associated cells.

Nerve cells have a very special characteristic; they are able to conduct impulses. That means that a nerve cell has electrical properties. In order for a nerve cell to exhibit these electrical properties, the cell membrane itself must then exhibit special properties. What makes a nerve cell different from all other cells is the nerve cell has the ability to manipulate these electrical properties. The nerve cell manipulates these properties via the manipulation of a net flow of charges across the cell membrane of effector targets or other neurons. The cell membrane of a nerve is a lipid bilayer that sequesters ions. Na+ and Cl- are maintained at a higher concentration outside the cell. This sequestration of ions leads to what is termed the resting membrane potential. This resting neural potential is due to the interior of the cell being more negative than the outside of the cell. In a typical neuron, the resting membrane potential is approximately -70mV. The resting potential is maintained by the sodium-potassium pump. This pump is found within the plasma membrane and utilizes ATP to actively transport sodium out and actively transport potassium in. This arrangement maintains a sodium concentration outside the cell and a potassium concentration inside the cell.

In order for these modulations to occur, the membrane utilizes ion channels to allow the flow of ions from interior to exterior and visa versa. These ion channels have conformational changes that allow the flow of ions through the channel. Each ion channel is selective for a particular ion. Therefore, ion channels have a configuration that requires it to be a transmembrane protein or a transmembrane protein complex. It is the central pore of the protein cannel that is selective for the particular ion. The conformational states of the channel are "open" and "closed". When the ion channel is open, the ions that are specific for that channel are free to pass. When the channel is in the "closed" conformation, the selected ions are prevented from flowing. The channels change conformation because of changes in the electrical or chemical environment. Many channels are able to rapidly alter the conformational states while others require a refractory period during the change from one conformational state to another. This refractory state may last only milliseconds between the open and closed positions.

Channels are classified according to the ions that pass through them, sodium, potassium etc. Channels are also classified according to what makes the conformational changes occur. If the channel is responsive to neurotransmitters (chemicals), then they are called ligand gated ions channels. When the appropriate neurotransmitter binds to its receptor on the membrane, it then produces a conformational change to allow the selected ions to flow. If the ion channel is responsive to differences in the voltage differences across a membrane, the channel is called a voltage gated ion channel. The changes in the membrane potential come from a local group of channels so that there may be distinctive zones for the hyperpolarization or the depolarization of the membrane. The term hypopolarization is when the membrane potential moves in the negative direction, thus becoming more negative. This situation would indicate an increase in the difference of the membrane potential. Depolarization is the term used when the difference across the membrane is reduced, moving closer to zero.

The situation of a variable membrane potential makes possible two types of membrane potential change. One is the graded potential change. In this graded potential, the value can be variable. The variability is dependent upon the intensity and the duration of the ion channel position, open or closed, and the initial membrane potential. These graded potentials are the result of opening one kind of ion channel, or could possibly result from the opening/closing of many different kinds of ion channels. It will gradually return to the resting membrane potential. This return is a gradual decay due to the changes in the ion channels, either opening or closing. In the other situations, an action potential exhibits a very explosive and large depolarization with repolarization that will follow. This action potential has a predictable and reproducible shape. The action potential is the result of the opening and closing of sodium and potassium channels. These channels are voltage gated and are found on the axon. As the action potential is propagated along the axon, the repolarization re-establishes the resting membrane potential. It is the changes in the permeability of the membranes that becomes the basis of the reception, propagation and eventual transmission of electrochemical information within the cell.

The neuron has a function to be the information gatherer for the nervous system. Sensory information enters the nervous system via the environment directly. The process of induction is the manner that the nervous system employs to convert sensory input into a useable form. This useable form is electric or chemical in nature. This is the form that the nervous system is able to transmit within the system. The olfactory system is a good example of a receptor that has chemical activation. There are two types of receptors in olfaction, but both are stimulated by a chemical stimulus. The hypothalamus is another example of this type of receptor.

There is also a receptor that is activated by a mechanical stimulus, and they are called mechanoreceptors. They take a physical force that is applied to them and transform it into an electrical stimulus at the sensory neurons. This type of receptor is commonly found in the vestibular, auditory, and somatosensory system. Other receptor types are the nocioreceptors and thermoreceptors. The nocioreceptors are responsible for the transduction of pain while the thermoreceptors transduce temperature changes within the skin and the viscera.

The neuron has a second function, transmission of the information that it receives from the periphery. In order for this to occur, one neuron must communicate with another. Communication is achieved via synapses and neurotransmitters. The synapse is the physiologic location of this communication. It is where one neuron will exert its effect on a second neuron or a target cell. Synapses are categorized by the morphologic characteristics they present. Primarily, there are two classifications of synapses, chemical and electrical. Majority of the synapses found in the human nervous system are of the chemical type. A chemical synapse has some definite components; they are a presynaptic component, a synaptic cleft and a postsynaptic component. The synaptic cleft is commonly about 20-50 nm wide. Presynaptically, the component is the axonal bouton. Within the bouton are many mitochondria that provide the energy required for the production of the neurotransmitter and other metabolic processes. Contained within the presynaptic component are many vesicles containing the actual neurotransmitter to be released into the synaptic cleft. Under the electron microscope, the vesicles are gathered at particular sites called the active zones. It is at the active zones where the neurotransmitter will be released.

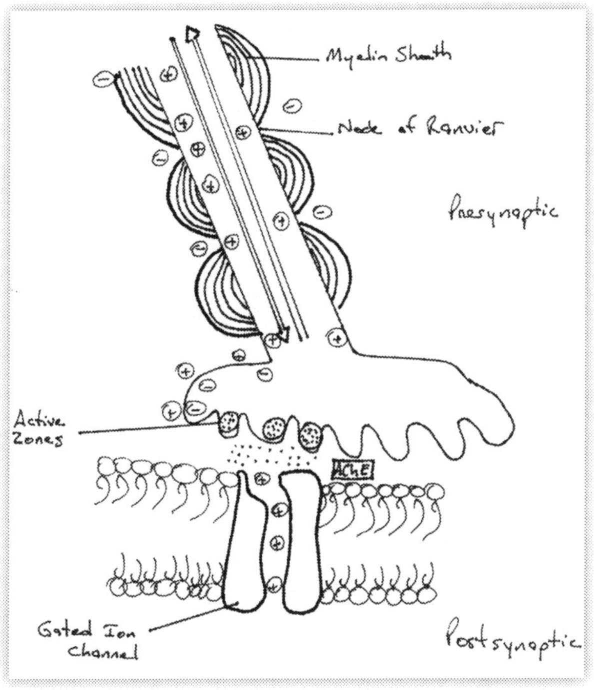

The release of the neurotransmitter from the presynaptic membrane active zone requires that an action potential be propagated along the axon to the axonal terminal. This action potential will produce a depolarization of the presynaptic membrane. The depolarization will in turn, activate calcium channels within the membrane. Upon activation, the calcium channels will open and allow calcium to increase its internal concentration. The increased intracellular calcium will cause the vesicles to fuse with the presynaptic membrane. After this fusion takes place, the vesicle will release the neurotransmitter contained within it. Each vesicle contains a fixed amount of neurotransmitter called quanta.

The neurotransmitter will diffuse into the cleft and across the cleft where a portion of the neurotransmitter will bind to a specific postsynaptic receptor. It is this binding of transmitter and receptor that will cause activation of an electrochemical change within the postsynaptic cell. Chemical synapses are unidirectional; they only transmit from the presynaptic to the postsynaptic cell. The strength of the postsynaptic response is directly proportional to the amount of neurotransmitter being released. Chemical synapses are classified by morphology as well. They are termed Gray's Type I and Gray's Type II. Gray's Type I have acetylcholine as the transmitter. The Gray's Type II synapse exhibits GABA as its transmitter. There are various other characteristics that will differentiate Gray's Type I from Type II. The Gray's type I synapse has a very asymmetric appearance when viewed under electron microscopy. This is due to the accumulation of the dense material found presynaptically that is not found post synaptically. These synaptic vesicles are large and clear, ranging in size from 30 to 60 nm. The Type I synapse itself has a larger synaptic cleft, approximately 30 nm wide and the synaptic region is long, ranging 1-2 um. This is in contrast with the type II synapses that have a symmetric appearance with the synaptic vesicles evenly distributed on the pre and postsynaptic membrane. The vesicles are pleiomorphic in shape. The type II synapse has a smaller synaptic cleft and a shorter synaptic region.

Even with the extensive understanding of the Gray's Type I and II synapses, there are vesicles that are seen with a dense core that are thought to contain serotonin or other neuropeptides. However, these vesicles are not represented in the Gray's categorization. Chapter 8 and 13 will deal further with the idea of synapses and neurotransmitters.

Glial cells are another type of cell in the nervous system. Glial cells are the most numerous cell type in the human nervous system. The function of the human brain is dependent upon the glial cell, even though the glial cell does not propagate an action potential. Glial cells do have processes that extend from the soma but these processes are not designed to receive or to transmit electric potentials. The function of a glial cell is one of structural support as well as maintenance of the internal environment of the nerve. The glia are called astrocyte, or oligodendrocytes, or microglia in the CNS. In the PNS, the correlative cell type is the satellite cell, or the Schwann cell and the macrophage.

Astrocytes are found throughout the CNS. The unique feature of the astrocyte is that it has "end feet" at the terminal aspect of the highly branched processes. It is the end feet that will form the protective barrier of the CNS. The glia limitians is a thin layer of these end feet that is located beneath the pia mater. This membrane has been termed the glial limiting membrane. This same type of protective layer of glial end feet is likewise extended around each and every blood vessel within the CNS. Within the CNS there are two differing types of astrocytes that help to create this protective barrier. Protoplasmic astrocytes are found within the grey matter of the brain. These astrocytes are different in shape from the fibrous astrocytes of the white matter. In order to separate them, identification of an intermediate filament protein called glial fibrillary acidic protein is chemically stained for. Glia also plays a substantial role in the developing nervous system. In the developing nervous system, they are radial glia, and their function is to lay down a framework that will guide neuronal migration. In the fully developed adult brain, it has been demonstrated that astrocytes are responsible for the secretion of several growth factors. These growth factors play a vital role in the support of a neuron. This is one reason that researchers believe to be the mechanism of astrocyte proliferation after CNS injury that results in loss of neural tissue. This proliferation will result in the formation of an astrocytic scar. It is this same property that may be the clue as to why majority of the CNS tumors are of astrocytic origin. In certain disease processes, the astrocyte is responsible for the secretion of cytokines. These cytokines are a regulator of the functioning immune system.

Another important function of the astrocyte is the buffer capacity that an astrocyte possesses. The astrocyte contains the same ion channels that other cells have and these channels allow for the uptake of ions like potassium. These ions are the byproduct of the generation of the action potential. Astrocytes have a function in the metabolism of neurotransmitters. The role of disposal of unutilized neurotransmitter falls upon the astrocyte. This is done within the synaptic cleft. A good example of this is seen in the neurotransmitter glutamate. This amino acid neurotransmitter is taken up by the astrocytes and then inactivated by enzymatic addition of ammonia that will yield glutamine. This end product is then released by the astrocyte only to be reconverted in to glutamate within the neuron's perikaryon. This metabolic pathway is one way that the nervous system is able to detoxify ammonia.

The brain is extremely sensitive to changes in the internal environment. Small chemical changes can have drastic effects possibly even lethal. One way for the environment to be controlled, the brain is protected by the blood brain barrier. This protective barrier is made up of tight junctions that create a seal of endothelial cells. This barrier prevents the free flow of ions and solutes. For this regulatory control, solutes must pass through the endothelial cells. Water, gases, lipid-soluble small molecules are able to diffuse through the endothelial cells with little difficulty.

There is a second mechanism present for the regulatory control of this environment that is the decreased number of pinocytic vesicles. Within the CNS, there are a dramatically reduced number of these vesicles present so that there is a reduction in the amount of nonspecific transport.

The second major type of glial cell is the oligodendrocyte. This cell type is found within both white and gray matter. The function of the oligodendrocyte is that of myelination. Oligodendrocytes are also seen lying adjacent tot neuronal cell bodies within the gray matter, but the functional role of this configuration is not well understood.

Microglia is the other glial cell type found in the CNS. Microglia developed from monocyte-macrophage cell lines. The function of a microglia cell is much like that of a macrophage, in that they are cellular scavengers. When tissue damage occurs, the microglia is activated and they will migrate to the site of injury, there they will phagocytes cellular debris. During tissue injury, these cells will exhibit proliferation as well as the astrocytes. The microglia is also responsible for the production and the release of cytokines like the interleukins. Since microglia is macrophage lineage cells, they act as antigen presenting cells as well. Because of this property, it is thought that they play a role in autoimmune diseases of the CNS.

The peripheral nervous system has a group of cells that would correspond to the glial cells of the CNS. These supportive cells are the satellite cell and the Schwann cell. In the PNS, the satellite cell surrounds the cell body of the neurons of the sensory and autonomic ganglia. Schwann cells provide the myelin cover of the axon in the periphery. The large and medium sized axons within the PNS are myelinated while the small diameter axons are unmyelinated. The term unmyelinated is misleading, as even the smallest diameter axons are ensheathed in the Schwann cell. There are differences in the myelin of the CNS and the PNS. In the myelin of the PNS there are pockets of remaining cytoplasm that are called Schmidt-lanterman clefts. These are not seen in the CNS. There is also a basal lamina that covers the external surface of the Schwann cell. It is thought that this structure helps in the stabilization of the Schwann cell during its formation of the myelin sheath. Each and every internode of the PNS is indicative of a single Schwann cell. This is in contrast to the structure of the CNS where one oligodendrocyte sends out great many processes that form the myelin sheath. In the PNS, external to the Schwann cell basal lamina, three layers of connective tissue cover peripheral nerves. These layers are the endoneurium, the innermost layer, the perineurium, which in the middle layer, and the epineurium, the outermost layer. The endoneurium is made of very thin Type III collagen fibrils. On inspection with EM, there are fibroblasts apparent within the individual nerve fibers. Each fascicle of axon is covered by the perineurium. This is a very distinct layer on EM. The perineurium is made up of concentric layers of fibroblasts that are flattened but most percicularly; they have retained the basal lamina with many pinocytic vesicles. These perineurium layers are connected via tight junctions to form a protective layer, much like the blood brain barrier of the CNS. The epineurium is covering the entire peripheral nerve. This is made of a dense connective tissue of Type I collagen fibrils. There are typical fibroblasts within this layer of the neural covering.

The vast majority of peripheral nerve tumors are of Schwann cell origin hence the name schwannoma. These are normally well encapsulated and usually not inclusive of the nerve fibers themselves. The discussion of neural regeneration is a very large subject and will be addressed in depth in chapter 24. A brief overview will be given but this is by no means all—inclusive.

It has been well established that the adult human nervous system is not something with a great regenerative capacity. This is especially true of the CNS. There are no neuronal precursor cells present in the CNS to allow for this replication process. These precursor cells are the stem cells. It stands to reason that if the nervous system is damaged via disease or trauma, the ability of the system to recover is not good.

In the PNS, if the axon is the only aspect of the nerve that is damaged, there is a regenerative capacity. This capacity is dependent upon the axonal cell body remaining completely intact. The prognosis of regenerative capacity is much better if the injury is one of a crushing nature and not a complete transection. In the CNS the astrocytic scarring negates any ability of the nerve to regenerate. Scarring is one reason for this inability to regenerate as well as the cytokines released during this astrocytic proliferation that may be responsible for the inhibition of any regenerative processes.

CHAPTER 5

DEVELOPMENT OF THE HUMAN NERVOUS SYSTEM

The human brain is an amazing structure. It is the control center of the human body. It is the basis of every thought, feeling, perception and movement that a human performs. This amazing structure weighs approximately 800g at the time of birth. By age 6, it has grown to 1,200g. Then by the time it has reached its adult size it will weigh 1,400g. The development of the human nervous system is a very complex process in every aspect. Development of the human nervous system begins in utero and continues to remodel through adulthood and as we now better understand, continues throughout the entire life of the human organism. The importance of this is in the dynamic state of the human nervous system as we develop. The speed with which this system develops is one reason for its susceptibility to injury, trauma, malnutrition or genetic error.

The basic building blocks of the human nervous system will have been completed by the sixth gestational week. The development of the nervous system now has the basics to make very rapid and dramatic developmental changes. During the second trimester, the major processes that occur are the cellular proliferation, and cellular migration. Both of these processes will continue until the full term. The process of myelination begins during the initial phases of development and will reach peak activity during the middle of the third trimester. This process will continue into adulthood as well. These are just two examples of this rapidly developing and dynamic state of the human nervous system.

The initial part of the fetal tissue to be identified as the nervous tissue is the tissue called the epiblast or some references will call it the embryonic disc. The embryonic disc is noted to appear during the end of the second week of gestation. The embryonic disc is composed of ectoderm, mesoderm, and endoderm. The neuroectoderm is a specialized part of the ectoderm. Its importance comes from the manner it will give rise to the brain, spinal cord and peripheral nervous system. During week three of the gestation, the process of gastrulation begins. Evidenced now on the dorsal surface of the embryonic disc will be the beginnings of the primitive streak. This primitive streak will project from the primitive node (Hensen's node). In order for the development to continue as it will there is a new molecule that comes into play within the nervous system, the Cell Adhesion Molecule (CAM). The CAM's primary function is to promote the binding of the primitive neuroepithelial cells into defined structural components. The primitive streak will be a point of direction regulation of the neuroepithelial cells. Some cells will pass through the primitive streak and differentiate into the intraembryonic endoderm and mesoderm. Other cells will pass through the primitive streak and differentiate into the notochord. For this differentitation to continue, the neuroepithelial cells must pass through the primitive streak and continue in a rostral direction. During this same timeframe, the ectoderm that was identified earlier will begin to thicken and form the basis of the neural plate. These cells are spindle shaped and will continue to elongate. This concurrent process is of primary importance in the developing human nervous system as it marks the irreversible specificity of the developing human nervous system. The bulk of the human nervous system will be differentiated from this set of developing cells. This neural plate will be completed by week 3 of gestation.

In this cellular migration, the cells that will differentiate into the head will project rostrally as mentioned previously from the primitive knot as a thickening of cells located between the endoderm and the ectoderm. This projection will contain a lumen that is also called the notochordal canal and is seen to project caudally with opening into the amniotic cavity as the primitive knot. As differentiation of this structure continues, the primitive knot will become the neurenteric canal. The differentiation of the nervous tissue cells as they migrate from the centrally located prochordical plate and the primitive streak will be in a lateral and rostral-caudal direction. This means that the rostral aspect of the developing embryo is further along in development than the caudal aspect of the embryo. Even at this early developmental stage, the rostral aspect of this fetal tissue is larger and termed the presumptive brain while the caudal aspect is thinner and is considered as the spinal portion of the developing nervous system.

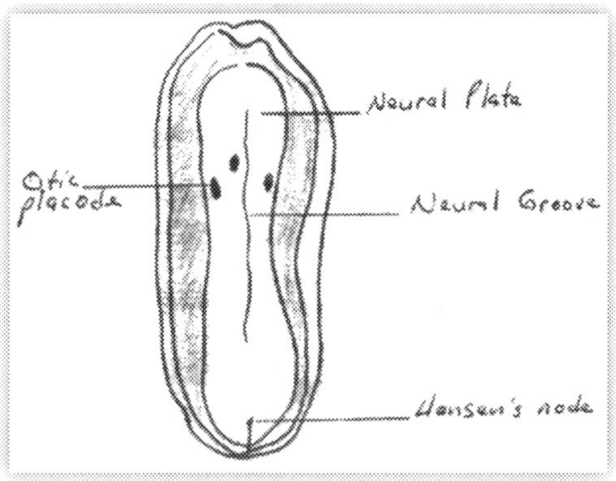

In general terms, the embryo is going to continue to elongate in a caudal direction. This means that the 14 somite stage has been reached at this time and the brain region is now developed into a "pore" like structure that contains an anterior and a posterior neuropore. These neuropores are important landmarks. Special cells will migrate away from the neural tube and the overlying ectoderm to form the neural crest. This differentiation is very complex as the early neural tube pseudostratified columnar epithelium will become the germinal or matrix cells. These germinal or matrix cells will then very quickly proliferate and will eventually produce the neuroblasts and the glioblasts.

Neurulation, primary and secondary neurulation is the term for this process of CNS development and differenttion. This process of neurulation is brought about due to the morphologic changes in the neuroblasts, immature and dividing future neurons. These cells become elongated and are seen to lie at 90 degrees to the dorsal surface of the neural plate. Cells designated as microfilaments are responsible for the elongation and the orientation of the cells. If there is an exposure to colchicine, that exposure will prevent neurulation from occurring. This exposure will lead to depolymerization of the microtubules will increase the likelihood of congenital defects. Exposure to cytochalasin will likewise lead to the inhibition of neurulation because of the inhibition of the contraction of the microfilaments. In previous discussion, there are two neurulation processes that the cell undertakes; primary neurulation and secondary neurulation. The primary neurulation is responsible for the development of the brain and the spinal cord while secondary neurulation is responsible for the development of the sacral and coccygeal regions of the spinal cord. Neurulation involves the development of the CNS from a hollow tube that is called the neural tube.

In primary neurulation, the neural plate will show thickening at the lateral edges. The proliferation of the lateral aspects of the neural plate will continue as structures termed, the neural folds. The initial thickening will occur at day eighteen of gestation. During this process of neurulation, the neural crest will pinch off and it will remain independent of the neural tube and the ectoderm. These neural crest cells will eventually differentiate into the dorsal root ganglia, sensory roots, the cranial root ganglia and the autonomic nerve ganglia parasympathetic and sympathetic motor neurons. This developmental milestone is important as it marks the time when the spinal dorsal root ganglia arrange in early somite formations. There will be concurrent development of the vertebral column structures and some of the cells will migrate ventrally to begin differentiation into the ventrally located neural system. Ventrally migrating cells will form the mesenteric ganglia, the celiac ganglia and the paravertebral ganglia. The developing Schwann cells and the satellite cells will share origins from the neural crest cell lineage as well as the sensory ganglia of CN V, VII, IX and X.

It is important to note that the schwann cells are not only of neural crest origins as there are some that will differentiate from the ventral and basal aspects of the neural tube and migrate as the peripheral nervous system will project and differentiate.

When the discussion of the development of the adrenals (suprarenal glands) comes about, it is important to understand that they have the same origins as the neural structures. It will become apparent at this point how those origins are evidenced. There will be a budding off of some of these structures as ventrally migrating cells that will become the chromaffin cells of the adrenal medulla. Through the differentiation of these cells and the migration of these cells from the neuroepithelial tissue, it is clear how the origins are alike.

By day twenty, the neural folds will begin to join together and fuse permanently. This fusion takes place in a predictable manner, the initial fusion will happen at the dorsal midline. This initial point of fusion will become the cervical region; the fusion will migrate in a rostral and caudal manner. As this process of fusion of the neural folds continues, the interior of the tube stays hollow. This is the neural canal and it is filled with amniotic fluid from it openings into the amniotic cavity rostrally and caudally. The openings will close at differing times of gestational age. The anterior neuropore, which is rostrally located, will close at day 24 while the posterior neuropore will close at day 26 of gestation.

At a point during the fourth week of gestation, the anterior neuropore will close with concurrent rapid proliferation of neural tissue in the cranial region. This is a period of very rapid tissue development. Prior to the anterior neuropore's closure, the rapid proliferation of neural tissue is faster than that of the remaining structures. The differential in growth means that there must be some mechanism for the neural tissue to fit in the space provided. The process of packaging the brain begins with the early prochordal plate being folded under the tissue of the forebrain.

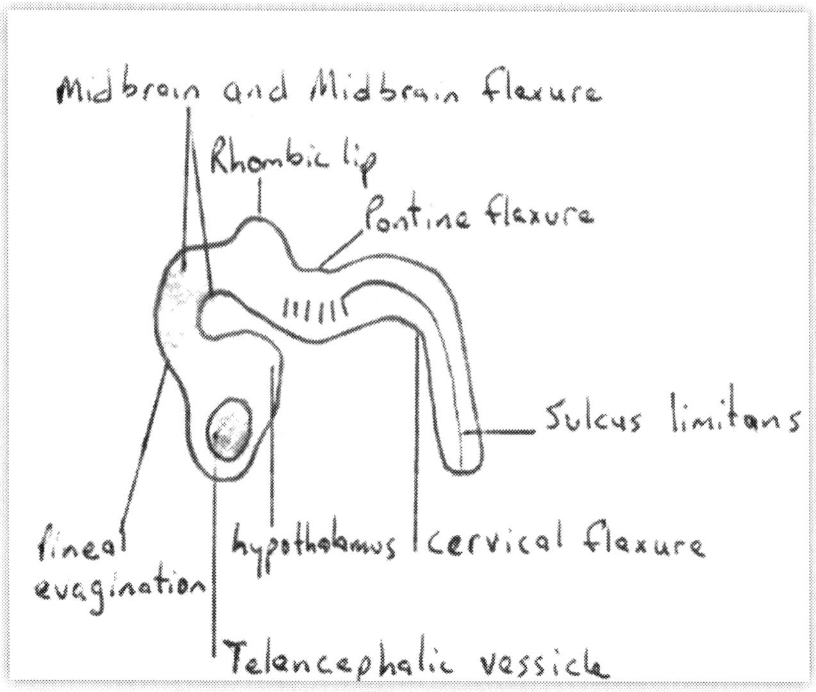

These tissues will produce the buccopharyngeal membrane as it continues in its development. This packaging of tissue will make it necessary to produce additional folds to accommodate the growing and developing brain mass. This is a very important aspect for the developing neural tube as compromise of the packing will elicit developmental problems. To accommodate the developing tissue, the neural tube will continue to "flex' or bend to produce folds, thus increasing the space available. The neural tube will flex in three principle locations, the initial ones will be the concurrent developing cervical and midbrain /mesencephalic flexures. These flexures will produce a ventral concavity that will be in stark contrast to the final neural tube flexure that will have a dorsal concavity, the pontine flexure. It is important for the medical student to understand the spacing discussed, as the cervical and the midbrain flexures are produced when the embryo is only 6 mm in length while the pontine flexure is produced when the embryo is 11-13 mm in length. If in the development of the neural tube, these flexures do not occur, there will be severe ramifications on the further development of the nervous system.

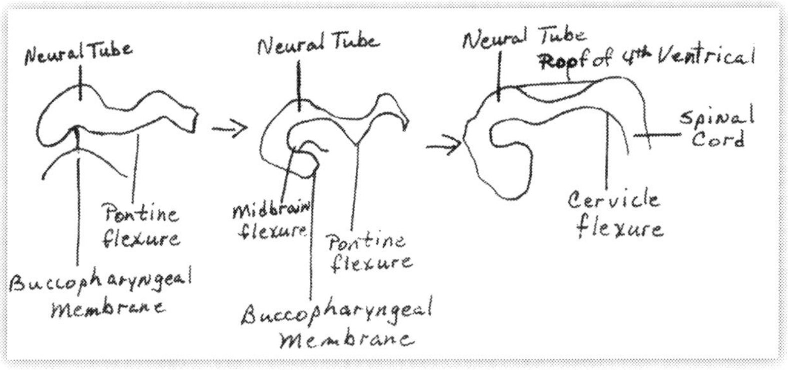

During this period of rapid proliferation and after the flexures noted above are produced, the three primary brain vesicles are formed. These are the proencephelon or the forebrain, the mesencephelon or midbrain, and the rhombencephelon or the hindbrain. Rostrally, the prosencephalon is found as a large mass of tissue. The prosencephalon will differentiate into the telencephelon and the diencephalon. Posterior to the prosencephalon, the mesencephalon is found at the midbrain flexure. More posterior, the rhombencephalon is found along with the now caudal myelencephelon as it is demarcated by the pontine flexure. The rhombencephalon will differentiate into the hindbrain while the myelencephalon will differentiate into the medulla.

PRIMARY DIVISION WITH THE EMBRYONIC NEURAL TISSUE

PRIMARY DIVISION	SUBDIVISION	FINAL STURCTURE
Prosencephalon	Telencephalon	Cerebral Cortex Basal Ganglia
	Diencephalon	Dorsal Thalamus Hypothalamus Epithalamus Ventral Thalamus
Mesencephalon (Midbrain)	Mesencephalon	Tectum Tegmentum Cerebral Peduncles

Rhombencephalon	Metencephalon	Cerebellum Pons
	Myelencephalon	Medulla

During the fifth week of gestation, these three primary vesicles will further develop into five secondary brain vesicles. The rhombencephelon or hindbrain will further develop into the meylencephelon and the metencephelon at the pontine flexure. This is also known as a dorsal flexure. The mesencephelon will remain unchanged. The proencephelon or the forebrain will develop into the diencephelon and the telencephelon. This development is the result of a budding off from the proencephelon. The development of the telencephelon is from a dorsal and caudal expansion of the bud. The buds are separated from the diencephelon by the telencephalic flexure.

Neuroanatomists will describe the process of the development of the forebrain as central induction. The primary structures of the forebrain will develop in the second month of gestation. Facial structures are forming from the mesoderm at the same time. This is why forebrain deformities are seen with concurrent facial abnormalities. Understanding the development of the nervous system, will help understanding the deformities and subsequent pathologies associated with maldevelopment. Anterior neuropore closure will produce a pair of outpouchings from the anteroventral lateral wall of the forebrain. These two outpouchings are defined as the optic vessicles. Initially, these vessicles are hollow and will migrate towards the thickening ectoderm to eventually produce the anatomic eye. Formation of the eye is derived from the invagination of the ectoderm producing the lens vessicle and the optic cup. It is the complex of surrounding tissue along with the lens vessicle and the optic cup that will differentiate into the finalized eye. The optic stalk which is the connection between the optic vessicle and the diencephalon will differentiate as the retina begins its formation. This will close off the connection between the diencephalon and the central cavity of the diencephalon / forebrain and the optic vessicle replacing it with what will be the eventual optic nerve fibers. The central cavity of the diencephalon will differentiate and become the third ventricle.

The telencephelon produces the telencephalic or cerebral vesicles. This differentiation is seen at the 5th week of gestation. The telencephalic vessicles are seen as outgrowths from the dorsolateral aspect of the maturing diencephalon. This growth is accelerated during months 4 and 5 in fetal development. This is in comparison to the remainder of the brain as the telencephalon is rapidly differentiating. These vessicles will differentiate into the eventual cerebral hemispheres and the basal ganglia. These two entities will compose the telencephalon. The walls of the telencephalic vessicles become thinned but the surface area rapidly expands. The majority of the growth is seen as an increase associated with the proliferation of the basal ganglia. The explanation for this disparity of growth is important and it is due to the three dimensional growth of the basal ganglia versus the two dimensional growth pattern of the hemispheres. The adult insula (island of Reil) is just beginning to develop and is seen as a small portion of the ventral telencephalon. In addition to the basal ganglia and the hemispheres, the formation of the ependymal cells is now able to be observed. The tissue origins of the hemispheres and the basal ganglia differ as the hemispheres have their origins in the neuroblasts that migrate through the mantle layer and move out to the marginal (outer) layer, while the neuroblasts that have congregated along the telencephalic vessicles will form the basal ganglia. These cells are found to lie along the base of the telencephalic vessicles.

This development of the ependymal cells is important as they are the production units of the cerebrospinal fluid that is required for the nervous system to continue to develop. The importance of these cells does not stop at birth; rather the importance of the fluid that is produced by these cells is seen as shifting duties and providing an environment that is maintained within a narrow range of variables. The ependymal cells and the position that they occupy is important for additional reasons as they are going to be pushed into an expanding sheet by the differential growth patterns discussed above. The development of the rapidly growing neural crest cells that constitute the basal ganglia will push into the sheet as if to be draped by the sheet. It is this pushing of the basal ganglia into the ventricle that will eventually form the inferior horn of the lateral ventricle. The telencephalic vessicles have a roof that is lined with the ependymal cells and it is of a configuration that in the early development is in communication with the third ventricle. The vessicles will communicate with the third ventricle as it establishes the foramen of Monro. The structural arrangement is important as the differentitation of these cells will continue into adult life. The anterior aspect of the foramen of Monro is in contact with the lamina terminalis and the posterior aspect of the foramen will be in contact with the thalamus. The inferior aspect of the foramen of Monro is in contact with the hypothalamus and the superior aspect is in contact with the roof of the diencephalon. These arrangements will become important and evident as the brain continues in its development. It is at this point that the hemisphere is now able to visualize the frontal, temporal, parietal occipital lobes and the insula. The insula will be covered by the neopallium or the hemisphere cortex to its position under the opercula. This orientation is important as it will lead to the formation of the lateral or the sylvan fissure from the failure of the frontal, parietal opercula and temporal operculum to fuse.

In the adult, the cerebral cortex, subcortical white matter, internal capsule, olfactory bulbs and tract, amygdala, and the hippocampus are all results of the final differentiation. The diencephelon will form the thalamic nuclei and the optic cup. The optic cup will eventually become the optic nerve and the retina. When the embryo attains a size of approximately 11.8 mm, the outpouchings of the diencephalon will become visualized, although not easily visualized until the embryo reaches approximately 16 mm in length. These outpouchings will then further differentiate into the thalamic subdivisions of the diencephalon. The dorsal thalamus, the subthalamus, the hypothalamus and the epithalamus will come to compose the mature thalamus in the adult brain. The wall of the third ventricle will be compressed to a very thin void as the surrounding neuroblasts continue to rapidly proliferate. The thalamic subdivisions will show the most rapid growth and because of this rapid growth they will be easily visualized and easily demonstrated as it abounds the third ventricle. The intimate relationship of the thalamus and the neopallium will develop in a concurrent pattern and it is because of this concurrent growth that we see such intimate interconnections between them in the adult brain.

In the development of the brain, the cerebral hemispheres will form communication pathways and these pathways will relay intricate information through many aspects of motor and sensory function. In the developing brain this presents a very unique structural problem as the developing ependymal tissue provides a substantial barrier to the growth of the pathways. Even though the ependymal layer is a single layer at this point, the nervous tissue cannot pierce this tissue layer. The neurons must look for a piggyback mechanism then to bridge into the opposite hemisphere. The tissue used as this piggyback is the lamina terminalis. Structurally, this is the only possibility as it is continuous with the choroid fissure of the opposite hemisphere through the roof of the third ventricle. This is the initial development of the commissural fibers. Development of the commissural fibers follows a pattern of oldest develops first. Therefore, the hippocampus is the first projection of fibers, and the projections are as the fornix. These fibers will migrate rostrally to the lamina terminalis following the hippocampus and the choroid fissure. These fibers will develop into the dorsal commissure as they project to the opposite hemisphere and final differentiation is as the hippocampal commissure. This pattern of rapid growth will produce a Caudally directed displacement of the corpus callosum from the lamina terminalis into the fornix. Concurrently, the hippocampus is going to be pushed medially into the forming temporal lobe. This deviation of the fibers in development will result in some fibers remaining dorsal to the corpus callosum and those fibers will differentiate into the medial and the lateral longitudinal striae of Lancisi and the indusium griseum. The corpus callosum continues to grow rapidly and this growth will displace the hippocampal commissure caudally and the fornix will be displaced rostrally. During this process of rapid growth there will be a release of the fornix from the corpus callosum that will be the rationale behind the medial wall of the third ventricle. As the corpus callosum continues to develop and grow posteriorly the great transverse cerebral fissure will develop and become evident.

The internal capsule is a C shaped structure that is found packed between the thalamus and the basal ganglia. Anatomically, the internal capsule will divide the basal ganglia into the globus pallidum and the putamen and the caudate nucleus. This is a very important differentiation as the anterior aspect of the frontal lobe will send projections into the anterior limb of the developing internal capsule. The projections to the lenticulothalamic aspect of the internal capsule will extend from the posterior frontal lobe and the parietal lobe. These fibers will pass the body of the lentiform nucleus, the thalamus and the caudate nucleus in creating this lenticulothalamic portion of the internal capsule. The retrolenticular portion of the internal capsule is composed of fibers of the occipital lobe projections while the sublenticular aspect of the internal capsule is composed of projections from the temporal lobe. The proximity and the inter-relations of these amalgamations of tissue explain the devastating nature of a malformation or damage within them.

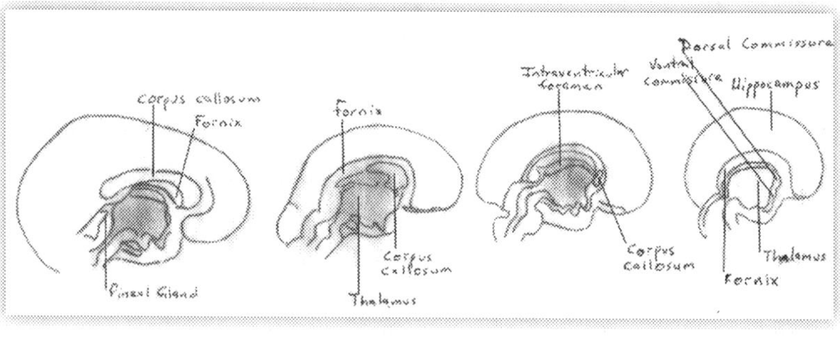

Secondary neurulation is the development of the sacral and coccygeal aspects of the developing spinal cord. As one looks at the structural configuration of the spinal cord from its inception on through the adult terminal differentiation, there are in many aspects very little changes apparent. In the spinal cord, the developing cord is produced from two major zones of proliferation, the alar plate and the basal plate. Once the process of differentiation and proliferation commences, development of the spinal cord and its associated structures, the intervertebral disc and the nerve roots seen at each corresponding level are now ready to begin maturation and continued proliferation. The anterior neuropore is known to close at approximately the 30th day of gestation. This closure is not the same on the posterior aspect of the neural tube. This separation in timing is the basis for the development of the spinal cord. The closure of the posterior neuropore is not evidenced until after the completed differentiation of the mesoderm from the primitive streak. This secondary neurulation is initiated at day 20 and will continue until the forty-second day of gestation. During this development, the caudal eminence will form. This will become evident as a mass just caudal to the caudal termination of the neural tube. This mass will enlarge and eventually cavitate. The caudal mass will eventually join with the neural tube. The cavity of this eminence will eventually join with the neural canal as well and become the basis of the spinal cord as it is attached or projected from the more rostral aspects of the developing brain. The cells of the alar plate will continue to differentiate as the dorsal aspect of the neural tube while the basal plate cells will continue to differentiate in ventral aspect of the neural tube. As differentiation continues, these zones will produce the dorsal horn from the alar plate zone cells and the posterior or dorsal horn by the basal plate zone cells. It is early in the developing embryonic tissue that the pneumonic: DAS VEM (Dorsal—Afferent-Sensory Ventral—Efferent-Motor) is identified. Anatomically, these zones are defined by an almost imaginary tract of tissue, the sulcus limitians. At this point in the developing embryo, the sulcus limitians is difficult to visualize. As the spinal cord differentiates and matures, the sulcus limitians will become easily observable and an important anatomic landmark.

This segmentation of rhombomere levels is structurally how we develop cranial nerve motor nuclei. The termination of the dural sac in the adult is at the level of S3. The manner that the spinal cord lengthens is extremely important as well. The developing spinal cord will differentiate and grow by having a permanent attachment point and in effect stretching out the cord in length. The change in position is not with the attachment of the cord, but rather the termination point of the cord. This anatomic point of connection is called the filum terminale.

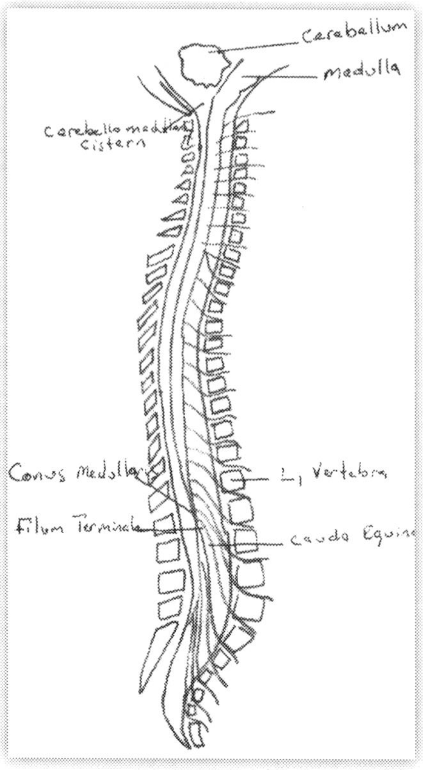

This is a fibrous tissue the anchors the spinal cord to the internal aspects of the vertebral canal. As a result of the growth differential, the coverings of the spinal cord must provide a variable growth pattern so as to keep in unison with the vertebral canal. The evidence of the variable position of the cord is seen clearly when the position of the nerve roots are visualized. The manner that the cervical roots exit the spinal cord will vary tremendously from those at the sacral level and the lumbar levels. In the cervical spinal cord, the nerve roots will exit the spinal cord in a position that is perpendicular to the cord, where the position of the adult lumbar and sacral roots will compose the cauda equina of the spinal cord and will exit several levels superior to the innervated areas. This separation of position is noted once the embryo reaches approximately 200 mm. This is called segmentation and it is a property that is not unique to the spinal cord. The hindbrain demonstrates segmentation as well. The segmentation of the spinal cord is due to the pattern of somite formation from the mesoderm. The axons of the motor neurons will exit and project into the anterior aspect of the corresponding somite and begin the segmentation of the spinal motor nerves. These cells will join with other cells from the neural crest and form the dorsal root ganglia. Anatomically, the sensory component of the dorsal root ganglia will project from the dorsal root ganglia and follow the motor nerve. The hindbrain produces its segmental organization from the Rhombomeres.

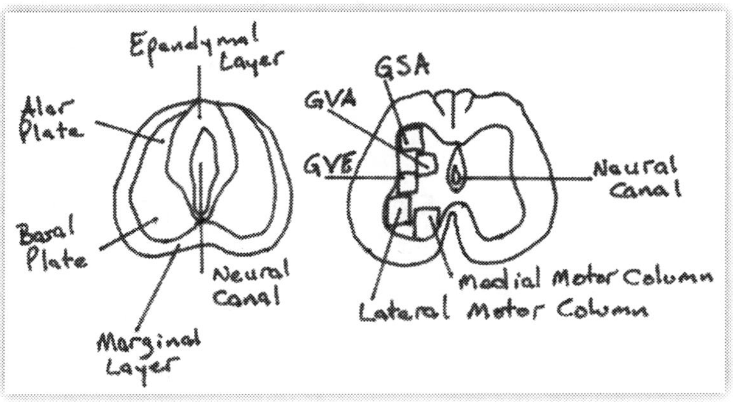

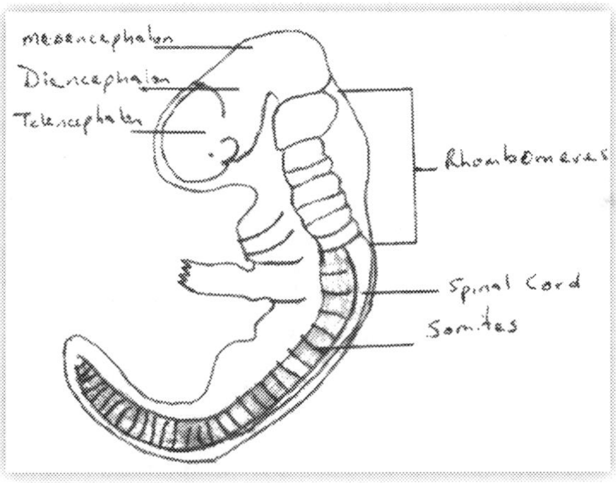

As a brief explanation, the ventricles are a very complex system that develops concurrently with the other aspects of the brain. The telencephalic vesicles will become the lateral ventricles and the diencephalic cavity will differentiate into the third ventricle. The forth ventricle will develop from the rhombencephalic cavity. The cerebral aqueduct of Sylvius develops from the mesencephalic cavity. This is the cavity that will connect the third and the fourth ventricle. This is a small opening 0.5 mm in diameter and as such is a common point of blockage of the ventricular system. The common anomaly is atresia or failure to develop. This is a common congenital developmental problem. The intraventircular foramina of Moro, develops from the openings of the lateral ventricles. This entire system is lined with ependymal cells, and a thin covering of pia mater. The layer of connective tissue is penetrated by blood vessels to form the basis of the choroid plexus. The foramen of Magendie and the foramen of luschka are openings that arise from the roof of the fourth ventricle. These are paired and are responsible for the passage of the CSF into the ventricular space from the lateral and the fourth ventricles.

The cavity of the forebrain will elicit the first and the second ventricles. These ventricles or cavities will differentiate further into the lateral ventricles. These lateral ventricles are easily identified and project as outpouchings from the most anterior aspect of the neural tube. Immediately posterior to the two lateral ventricles will be the third ventricle. This non-paired ventricle is located in the midline. The third ventricle is connected to the lamina terminalis and provided a conduit for the communication with the two lateral ventricles via the interventricular foramen of Monro. The lateral ventricles provide a framework for the development of the diencephalon and the remaining cerebral hemispheres. The lateral ventricles are seen with one in each hemisphere of the cerebrum. The shape that is identified in the mature adult of the lateral ventricles are present as the child brain develops in part due to the manner the ventricles are themselves formed. The drawing of the ventricles anteriorly, will provide this shape of the elongation of the initial “C” shape. The six (6) components of the lateral ventricle are; the anterior horn, the body, the antrum (containing the glomus), the inferior and posterior horns. The septum pellucidum and the fornix are known to provide boarders for the developing lateral ventricle and will remain throughout the adult life. The corpus callosum and the caudate nucleus with the thalamus will provide the floor of the lateral ventricle while the hippocampus and the amygdala will provide the ventral border.

The peripheral nervous system is derived from the neural crest cells. This development of the peripheral nervous system is complex and will continue into adulthood. The origin of the neural crest cells comes from the lateral edges of the neural plate. These cells will detach from the neural plate and then migrate to the lateral aspects of the region. There they will attach themselves to the spinal cord and the developing brain. There are two neuronal cell types that will develop from this tissue: the pseudounipolar cell and the multipolar cell. The ganglia of cranial nerves 5, 7, 8, 9 and 10 will receive tissue contribution from the placodes. The placodes are special epidermal cells.

The pseudounipolar nerve cells are sensory in nature. They develop from neuroblast cells. Individual neuroblast cells will produce a peripheral process and a central process. The peripheral process innervates the target tissue, while the central or proximal process that will enter into the brainstem or the spinal cord. The neural crest cells initially are of a fusiform shape and apolar but will alter the structure as they develop. The structural changes consist of a fusion of several processes near the cell body to yield the eventual T-shaped structure. It is this structural change that is the reason behind the name of the pseudounipolar neuron. The cell body of this cell is found in the dorsal or posterior root ganglia. This structure is found situated next to the spinal cord. In the dorsal root or posterior root, the cells are of neural crest origin as stated earlier. The spinal nerve has a corresponding segment called the somite. These are the segmentation of the nervous system in the developing embryo. As the somites grow to form portions of the body's connective tissue as well as musculature, the peripheral processes of the corresponding dorsal root ganglia will grow distally. There are a group of proteins responsible for the growth of the distal processes. These are fibronectin and laminin. These matrix molecules are found to contain a specific amino acid sequence of arginine—glycine—aspartate, otherwise known as the RGD sequence. It is this sequence that is recognized by another protein called integrins. Integrins are located on the surface of the neural crest cells. These proteins are thought to be responsible for the growth of the peripheral processes of the pseudounipolar cells and guide them to the eventual target tissue. Demonstration of this segmental development is seen in the dermatomes and myotomes used in the diagnostic scheme of pathologic states.

STRUCTURES DERIVED FROM NEURAL CREST CELLS

NEURAL ELEMENTS

dorsal root ganglia
sympathetic chain / paravertebral ganglia
enteric ganglia
Parasympathetic ganglia of CN 7, 9, 10.
Sensory ganglia of CN 5, 7, 8, 9, 10.

NON-NEURAL ELEMENTS

Schwann cells
Melanocytes
Odontoblasts
Satellite cells of peripheral ganglia
Cartilage of the pharyngeal arches
Ciliary and pupillary muscles
Chromaffin cells of the adrenal medulla
Pia and arachnoid meningeal layers

They are also found within the sensory cranial nerve ganglia. There are exceptions to this situation, namely the mesencephalic nucleus of the trigeminal nerve. This exception in structure is due to the failed migration of these cells with the neural crest cells.

There are cranial nerve ganglia that are also derived from the neural crest cells and the placode cells. These ganglia are composed of pseudounipolar cells as well. The ganglia are the Trigeminal or semilunar, the Geniculate, and the ganglia of the glossopharyngeal ganglia,(both the superior and the inferior). The jugular and the nodosa ganglia are likewise derived from the neural crest cells. The structural distribution of these ganglia is such that the distal processes of these cranial nerves act as the sensory component and the proximal processes act as the cranial nerve nuclei within the brainstem.

There are still other cells derived from the neural crest cells. One such group of cells is the cells of the Visceral Motor system, specifically, the post-ganglionic sympathetic and parasympathetic neurons. In the adult, these neurons are of multipolar appearance but they do originate from the apolar neuroblasts. Many of these cells remain close to the site of origin in the form of the sympathetic chain ganglion. This structure can be found alongside the vertebral column. Still other cells will migrate to the aorta and form the sympathetic prevertebral ganglia. The rhombencephelon is the site of origin for the majority of the autonomic nerves that will innervate the digestive tract. These are the Meissner's and Auerbach's plexus. The autonomic innervation of the descending colon and other pelvic structures are also derived from the sacral cord during the secondary neurulation process.

Another important structure that is of neural crest derivation is the Schwann cell. These cells are responsible for the myelination of the nerves of the peripheral nervous system. As was stated earlier, the Schwann cells will migrate in segmental fashion following the peripheral processes of the peripheral nerve they protect.

The development of the central nervous system is somewhat different in its development. The neuroblasts that will eventually lead to the formation of the central nervous system originate at the luminal surface of the neural tube. These cells are of pseudostratified columnar epithelium subtype. During the days that will follow the neural tube will thicken and the cells will show a strange pattern of aggregation during this proliferation. They will cluster about the ventricular surface in such a manner as to leave the cell bodies oriented so that there is a zone of no cell bodies called the marginal zone, along the abluminal surface. During the differentiation process special glial cells, radial glia are responsible for the direction of migration. It is the radial glia that assists in the migration away from the luminal surface to produce what we call the intermediate zone. This zone of proliferative cells is found between the luminal or ventricular zone and the marginal zone. Once the cells have moved into the final position, they will begin to extend processes so that they can form connections between other neurons or target tissues. The processes are functional as they develop. Evidence if this is seen, as the dendrites are able to receive impulses from other developing cells. The axons are a different story. The axon is seen to exhibit a tip. This tip is called the axonal growth cone. This cone is responsible for the guiding of the axon through tissues to eventually reach its target. This is a structure that has come into more significance lately as a mechanism for the direction of neuronal growth following damage to the neuron. It has been demonstrated to be important in the process of neural sprouting.

Ironically, both the neuron and the glial cell appear to have the same developmental lineage. The theory is that the two cells seem to have the same precursor cell. The glioblastic cell lineage produces the likes of the radial glia, astroglia, and oligodendrocyte. This glioblastic lineage has three main branches that arise from it: Type I astrocyte progenitor, oligodendrocyte type II astrocyte progenitor or the O2A progenitor, and a radial glia progenitor. The radial glia cell is the only subclassification that does not remain into adulthood. The radial glia cell does something unusual; it continues to differentiate but in the course of this differentiation it will develop into a different cell form. This new cellular form is the astrocyte, ependymal cell or the tanycyte. The situation is different in the cerebellum and the retina. Radial glia will develop into Bergman glia or Muller glia. These cells will retain most of the characteristics of the original radial glia. The key to this differentiation appears to be the growth factors like platelet—derived growth factor, ciliary neurotrophic growth factor, and fibroblastic growth factor. These growth factors are secreted by neighboring cells (glia and neurons), and signal the cells adjacent to them to differentiate. Our understanding of these growth factors has expanded significantly in recent years as they have been the focus of multidisciplinary research teams for the broad impact that they have in our developing nervous system.

Development of the spinal cord is initiated from the caudal aspect of the neural tube. The neural canal is retained as the central canal of the cord. As mentioned earlier, the neuroblasts that produce the spinal cord neurons are themselves produced during week four (4) to week 20 of gestation. The cells will then move laterally and peripherally to form the four longitudinal plates. They will form two ventral plates and two dorsal plates. The ventral plates will be called the basal plates and the dorsal plates the alar plates.

The basal and the alar plates will be separated by a groove that will run longitudinally along the length of the entire cord. This groove is the sulcus limitans. It is contained inside the central canal within the lateral wall and is found separating the basal and alar plate bilaterally. The basal plate will differentiate into the ventral horn while the alar plate will differentiate into the dorsal horn. The intermediate zone of the adult spinal cord is formed by the interface between the alar and basal plates. Development of the basal plate will produce axons that will become the motor innervation to the peripheral structures. The basal and the alar plates will eventually develop into the gray matter of the spinal cord.

The ventral horn motor neurons innervate skeletal muscles and are therefore termed general somatic efferent or GSE cells. Lateral horn cells that project on to autonomic or visceromotor ganglia are called general visceral efferent or GVE cells. These two cell groups are referred to as the functional components of the spinal cord. The GSE and the GVE components are separate and yet distinct longitudinal columns within the gray matter. There are however differences in the length of each column. The GSE columns run the entire length of the cord while the GVE only extend from T1down through L2. This column has a specific name the intermediolateral cell column. Structurally, it picks up again and runs from S2 to S4 and it is now called the sacral visceromotor nucleus.

Neurons from the alar plate will receive the central processes of the developing dorsal root ganglion. If the peripheral nerve processes innervate the skin, receptors in the joint capsule, tendons, or muscles they are classified as General somatic afferent or GSA cells. If the processes will innervate the receptors in the visceral structures, these will then be classified as General visceral afferent or GVA cells.

During this development, each somite will again subdivide into three distinct structures. The sclerotome will form the vertebra. The dermatome will become the skin and the dermis. The myotome will become the muscular system. The dermatome and the myotome will be innervated by the dorsal and ventral roots of each corresponding spinal cord level. These roots will join to form the spinal nerve at the neural foraminia. The sclerotomes will eventually form intersegmental tissue. This is in direct contrast to the segmental nature of the sclerotome. This unusual situation develops because the vertebra comes from the joining of a caudal and a cranial half from adjacent sclerotomes. This is made possible because the sclerotome will split at each segment into a cranial and a caudal portion.

The spinal cord has a unique developmental sequence. It maintains its general shape from the third trimester until adulthood, but its physical relationship to the vertebral column is what drastically changes. The meninges, spinal cord and vertebral arches are all formed by the completion of the first trimester. At this point the spinal nerves formed as noted above, will exit at right angles to the long axis of the spinal cord. The sequence changes radically from this point on, the vertebral column will grow at a much faster pace than the fully developed spinal cord. This differing rate of growth has the result of pulling the spinal cord rostrally since it has a point of fixed attachment at the brainstem. The thin filum terminale is the membranous distal point of attachment. This point of attachment is found at the S2-3 level, while in the adult the spinal cord termination is at L1-2. It is this configuration that allows for the removal of CSF during a lumbar puncture to be removed at the L3-4 level with little worry of damage to the cauda equina. The portion of most lengthening is at the lower lumbar, sacral and coccygeal aspects. This pulling of the cord will produce the cauda equina. Myelination of the spinal cord is unique as well as the cervical segments of the spinal cord are seen to myelinate first. Myelination begins with the intersegmental fibers to the motor neuron.

The brainstem consists of the medulla oblongata or the meylencephelon, the pons or a portion of the metencephelon and the mesencephelon or the midbrain. As development proceeds, there are two changes that take place when the brain is viewed from a rostral-caudal manner. The first is the appearance of the cerebellum with the concurrent opening of the central canal as it adjoins into the fourth ventricle. These changes force the dorsal portion of the neural tube or the alar plate into a dorsolateral position. The second major change is the loss of the sulcus limitans, structurally. There are remnants of the structure in the floor of the fourth ventricle that will act as a landmark for anatomists and clinicians. The columnar development of the brainstem is similar to that of the spinal cord. The differences are found in the number of columns, there are six cell columns and seven functional components in the brainstem. Where there are only four columns in the spinal cord. The higher functions of the brainstem are believed to be the reason for this accounting change. These higher functions are the special senses. The special visceral afferent or SVA, the special visceral efferent or the SVE, and the special sensory afferent or the SSA are innervations that are unique aspects of the head. These columns may during continued development, fragment into separate nuclei. These nuclei will then retain the same functional components and generally will retain the same structural alignment.

The alar plate will primarily develop into sensory tissue. There will be five cranial nerve nuclei to develop from this alar plate; they are the spinal trigeminal nucleus, the principle sensory trigeminal nucleus, the solitary nucleus, the vestibular and the cochlear nuclei. The inferior olivary nucleus, the basilar pontine nuclei and the substantia nigra are also derived from the alar plate. There is confusion often as the peripheral fibers projecting from the vestibular and the cochlear nuclei also have origination in the otic placode. The spinal trigeminal nucleus and the principle sensory trigeminal nucleus receive GSA input via cranial nerves 5, 7, 9, and 10. The solitary nucleus receives input from cranial nerve 7, 9, and 10.

The basal plate is the origin of most motor fibers of the brainstem. Almost all the cell structure of the basal plate is formed from separate nuclei. The most medial column nuclei are GSE functional components and will innervate the muscles that have occipital somite origin or mesoderm tissue origin from around the eye cup. The nuclei are the hypoglossal the abducens the occulomotor and the trochlear nuclei. Moving laterally, the next column is of GVE function and will innervate visceral motor ganglia. These nuclei represented are the dorsal motor vagal, the inferior salivatory, the superior salivatory nucleus, and the Edinger-Westphal nucleus. Projections from these nuclei move through the vagal, glossopharyngeal, facial and occulomotor nerves. Moving more laterally, the most lateral and ventral column will innervate muscles of mesodermal origin, specifically the pharyngeal arches. Thus, they are of SVE functional componentry.

The nuclei that are derived from this column are the ambiguus, facial and trigeminal nucleus.

The segmental development of the brain has been shown to be in a variety of planes, dorsal-ventral and rostral-caudal. In the rostral-caudal segmentation of the developing rhombencephelon, there is a segmentation called rhombomeres. These are neuroblastic cells that are separated from each other by thin transverse bands of neuroepithelial cells. The cells of one rhombomere will produce only one motor nucleus. These rhombomeres do not move to adjacent rhombomeres, so they do not mix. The development of the sensory information will enter at the corresponding rhombomere. The other important function of the rhombomere is the activation of the genetic home box gene. This home box gene is the "master switch "of formation of large blocks of tissue.

The cerebellum has a very interesting origination, arising from the rhombic lip. The rhombic lip is a portion of the alar plate from the wall of the fourth ventricle. The rhombic lip is divided into two portions, the rostral portion that will form the cerebellum and the caudal portion that will make the inferior olivary nucleus, cochlear nuclei and the pontine nuclei. It is how the rhombic lip forms the cerebellum that is important in this developmental sequence. The rhombic lips will join dorsally to produce the fourth ventricle and thus form the cerebellar plate. At this time, the fissures that appear will continue to divide the cerebellum into the main lobes. One lobe the posterolateral fissure, will divide the cerebellar plate. It is the first fissure to form. Next will be the flocculonodular lobe and then the corpus cerebelli. The next fissure to develop in this sequence is the primary fissure and it is the dividing mark between the anterior and the posterior lobe. Failure of these fissures to develop will produce conjoining lobes ad therefore developmental aberrations. During continued cerebellar development, the appearance of additional fissures will continue to form the characteristic structure of the adult cerebellum.

As with the rest of the human brain, the cerebellar cortical development is from the migration of neuroblastic cells. The primordium of the cerebellum is composed of a ventricular zone. This zone is subdivided into an intermediate zone and a marginal zone. The second layer appears at the end of the first trimester. This layer is identified on the outer aspect of the marginal layer, and is called the external granular layer. At this time in the differentiation process the name of the intermediate zone changes to become the internal granular layer. The internal granular layer is responsible for the eventual formation of the purkinji cells and the Golgi cells. These cells have differentiated from the neuroblast cells within the internal germinal layer. Within the ventricular layer and extending outward are the radial glial cells that were discussed previously in the chapter. It is important to remember the function of these radial glial cells being responsible for the migration of the neurons during development. Experimental evidence has demonstrated the neuroblasts will follow the radial glia cells for the directional migration.

Contrary to the pattern of migration of the internal granular layer are the neuroblast cells of the external granular layer. These cells will migrate inward. Again, the radial glial cells are the directional leaders of the developing neuron. The inward migrating neuroblasts will differentiate into granule cells. Cells that will differentiate into stellate cells and basket cells of the molecular layer will originate in the external granule layer as well. These cells are found just external to the purkinji layer. There are numerous important functions associated with the differentiation of these layers of cells. The granule cells sprout axons that will eventually form synaptic connections with the Purkinji cell dendritic trees that project into the molecular layer. This is an imperative function, as without these connections, the dendrites will not continue with their development progression. The result of this loss of development is devastating for continued differentiation and sensory integration.

The alar plate is also the origination of the thalamus. This comes about from the differentiation of the alar plate into the diencephelon. This differentiation occurs at 4 weeks gestation. Completion is by the sixth week of gestation. By week six the epithalamus, the thalamus and the hypothalamus are evident as swellings within the wall of the third ventricle. Distinguishing each of the three swellings are the epithalamic sulci and the hypothalamic sulci. During continued development, the epithalamus remains very small.

The thalamus and hypothalamus on the other hand will continue to enlarge during this same period of rapid development. There is a special case of the joining of the hypothalamus and the thalamus during development that is necessary for proper neural circuit development. This is called interthalamic adhesion or Massa intermedia. This thalamic development will follow a similar pattern to the rest of the nervous system; neuroblastic cells will migrate along radial glia cells that have projected from the third ventricle. There is some difference in the final developmental pattern, in the thalamus; the first neurons that undergo final differentiation will migrate into the outer aspects of the thalamus to complete maturation. Structurally, this means that the geniculate nucleus is the first to develop and the dorsolateral nuclei are the last to develop.

The cerebral cortex will follow like differentiation patterns but there is a major difference that must be identified as well. The cortical neuroblasts will maintain connections to the ventricular and the pial surfaces. This will elicit a fusiform shape to the cell. The first cells to migrate leave the guiding radial cell and remain close to the ventricular surface. As layer after layer of the proliferating neuroblastic cells will force themselves along the radial glia cell to take up final position closer to the pial layer, the internal structures become more evident. In order to do this they must push through the preceding layers of proliferated cells. These layers of cells will form the cortical plate. The cerebral cortex is formed from the intermediate zone, subplate and the cortical plate. The subplate is a structure that will not remain into adulthood. Inspection of the area between the subplate and the ventricular layer is the area that will eventually become the white matter. This area will become void of neuronal cell bodies, leaving only glial cells. This pattern of development will leave the ventricular zone as a single layer of cells that will be the ependymal cells of the lateral ventricle of the adult nervous system.

CHAPTER 6

NEURAL CIRCUITS

The Human Nervous System is analogous to an electric circuit. It shares many of the same properties that a closed electric circuit system does. It exhibits resistance, capacitance, carries a defined voltage (interchangeable with potential), follows Ohm's law, has polarity, and has a resistor, insulator and many more parallels with those seen in electrical circuits. The driving force behind this electrical model is a chemical based origin of membrane potential. In the human nervous system, the electrochemical neural impulse is created by the voltage difference that is derived from the flow of ions across the neural membrane. It is the net flux of these ions that dictates if there is an action potential or not. This principle of ion flow or exchange is paramount in the activity of the entire system, for sending, receiving and integrating of neuronal imputs.

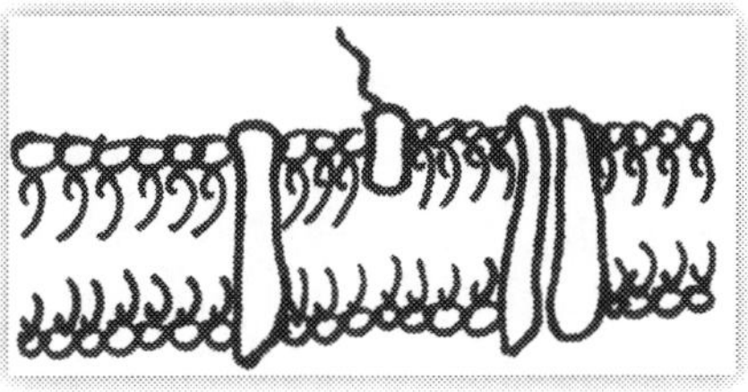

The neuron membrane has a basic structure of a lipid bilayer. This is a very important property for the neuron as it provides several functions. The main lipid component of the cell membrane is that of a phospholipid, the importance of this is the structure of the phospholipid and the polarity of the phospholipid. This polarity is what provides for the alignment that we see with the orientation of the polar head and the alignment of the hydrocarbon tail. In aqueous solution, the phospholipid will form micelles, spheres that have at the central core of hydrocarbons and the outer surface the polar heads. This is an orientation that has been demonstrated to be of the least energy expenditure versus any other configuration. The lipid bilayer provides a functional base with which the cell can function in the nervous system and within the internal environment of the body. This is no different than what we seen in other cells. The insulation component of the cell membrane is however a main property of the neuron that sets it aside from other cells of the human body. This hydrophobicity exhibited by the structure produces electrical capacitance. Capacitance of the thin cell membrane provides the separation of charge required to store the electrochemical energy to drive other aspects of the neuron's functional job. This structural arrangement is also a tremendous architectural design for the incorporation and attachment of the integral and transmembrane proteins that will provide the framework for the channels that will allow the flux of the ions across the capacitor that is the neuronal cell membrane. The most basic aspect of the structure of the lipid bilayer is the barrier that it provides to isolate and sequester ions, both within the cell and outside the cell. This lipid bilayer has also been demonstrated experimentally to provide a mechanism for cell communication and enzymatic activity. This is a very key component to the cell for many reasons. One major reason is the receptor function provided by the neuron's integral proteins. They are also a mechanism that the body uses for recognition, in other words they define the cell by labeling it. However, the main component for these integral proteins will be the ion channels that they will provide for the ions like: Na^{+}, Ca^{2+}, K^{+}, Cl^{-}. These channels will respond to the imbalances of the ions within and outside the cell. In the human neuron, the differential between the ion concentration within the cell and outside the cell is very dramatic, and is the basis for the drive that pushes the system.

Extracellular vs. Intracellular ion concentration

IONS	EXTRACELLULAR CONCENTRATION	INTRACELLULAR CONCENTRATION
Na+	120mM/L	12mM/L
K+	5mM/L	130mM/L
Cl^-	125mM/L	5mM/L
Ca^{2+}	2mM/L	0.0001mM/L

In the human nervous system, we talk of membrane potentials, action potentials and any perturbation of those baseline values. In order to understand the human nervous system, one must understand how this membrane potential is achieved and by what mechanism is this potential maintained or altered. In this section we will discuss the mechanism of the membrane potential, how it is established and deviated from. A neuron must provide some mechanism for the separation of the charges within the cell and outside the cell. This ability to separate charge is performed by the lipid bilayer membrane. This is the basic principle of the functioning of the system, keeping the inside of the neuron slightly more negative than the outside and then the reversals and restoration of these membrane potential or ion gradients. In the human nervous system we measure this change in millivolts (mV). In neuroscience we talk about this difference of ion position as a separation of charge that will result in a resting state or resting potential. The value assigned to this difference is considered to be a resting membrane potential of between -70 to -90 mV. In order for the system to function, there must be a mechanism available to produce very rapid changes in the membrane and then to return it to its baseline value. In terms of the nervous system this change is related to the flow of ions in and out of the cell, traversing the lipid bilayer discussed above.

Fortunately, we have a tool at our disposal to allow this function. The mechanism provides a simple yet dependable mode of transferring these ions both in and out of the cell. It also provides an ability to repeat the process millions of times throughout the life of us as beings. In our structure as human organisms, we produce proteins for many different reasons. One of the basic principles of this membrane potential is the rapid movement of ions across this lipid bilayer membrane. In order to achieve this goal, we utilize a transmembrane protein called an ion channel. These ion channels are able to allow flow of many ions through the openings in a very short period of time. These channels or pores are very selective for the ion that is allowed to pass through. Ion channels are available in open or closed states. The channels are able to be regulated or gated depending on several factors. With the selectivity being specific, and the flow restricted by that selectivity, the structure of the channel or pore must play a role in this process. This selectivity is provided by exclusion by charge and by size of the ion. This is how the term "voltage gated" or gated channel was derived. Ion channels do not normally conduct charges but in certain circumstances they are able to carry a small amount of charge. Channel selectivity for the charge is designed to allow the passage of cations while preventing the passage of anions. The mechanism may be from the steric hindrance of the interior of the aqueous pore of the channel or it may be from some other structural component. Secondary to the structural aspect of selectivity is the activation of the channel, being able to switch from an open or active stage to a closed or inactive stage. These ion channels then must have some mechanism of "activating or deactivating". The voltage gated channels demonstrate a collective architectural likeness, that of having the larger α subunit and a variable β subunit.

In the prototype sodium channel, there are four (4) domains of the α subunit (I, II, III, IV) that made up of six (6) membrane spanning segments of amino acids. There is a distinguishing sequence of the S segment peptide that delineates one from another. The S4 segment has been demonstrated by X Ray Crystal Fragment to contain positively charged R Side chains, further distinguishing each of the S subunits. These properties are common among the other cation channels as mentioned previously. This configuration is responsible for the actual pore that allows the flux of ions as described. It is also the characteristic that creates individual selectivity among channels. In other variants of the voltage gated channel there are connections between the six transmembrane helical structural domains made by hydrophophilic amino acids that demonstrate a flip flop pattern of arrangement with the polar aspect flipping from intracellular to extracellular alignment. Experimental evidence from cloning studies and sequencing studies have shown that the Na^+ channel coding sequence is much larger than that for the K^+ channel. The analysis work has shown a repeating sequence of amino acids within the six (6) transmembrane subunits that make up the channel. Each unit of the subunit is composed of sequences of approximately 250,000Kd. Even with this size of sequence, it is the protein folding capacity that makes the subunit ideal for its role in the channel structure. It has also been identified as the sequence in the similar domains of the K^+ and Ca^{2+} channels. With the advent of better analysis techniques, identification of the actual representation of the pore has been achieved. In the pores of the Na^+, Ca^{2+} and the K^+ channels, there has been identified a 20 amino acid domain (S5-S6 linker region) consistent in each channel type. The data is suggestive that this is actually the internal portion of the pore that produces the ion selectivity of the channel. Analysis of the region has shown a unique alignment of the amino acids. In the pore, it appears that there is a hydrophobic sequence that is set apart from a hydrophilic sequence every 3.5 residues. This will elicit the interaction with the shell of hydration of the ion as it is passing through the pore. In addition to the S5-S6 region is the S4 domain that has a similar task associated to it. The S4 domain contains the positively charged amino acid R side groups that occupy every third position to create an ion sensitive arrangement. It is this mechanism that is thought to be the activation trigger. Therefore if there is alteration in the sequencing or of the valance electron arrangement, the ability to provide adequate ion flow and change the ability of the neuron to respond to the stimuli presented.

Evidence of this property is demonstrated by electron microscopy and the alteration of charge as it relates to time. Experimental data from single cell recordings of the giant squid provided substantial data in the manner a cell separates charge. In the prototype experiments to understand the membrane behavior to ions British scientists Andrew Huxley, Alan Hodgkin and Bernard Katz described the behavior of the ion channels as they investigated them in the giant squid axon. As mentioned above, the transmembranous ion channel is a protein channel. These transmembranous channels are unique in structure, having the non-charged lipophilic amino acid side chains providing the stability for the channel. The variable numbers of ions allowed entrance and exit from the cell require variable transmembrane channels. The manner a channel becomes "activated" or "deactivated" is a variability of the channel itself. Neurons are described as having voltage sensitive gated channels. This is true for the basis sodium-potassium channel. In this traditional view of the nervous system, the potassium channel is the most basic and simple model to understand. The potassium channel provides for a single ion and activation state. The potassium channel has some variation but not the same as the sodium channel that will be discussed later. The potassium channel does contain a subsection of channels that display a delayed rectifier property. They obtained the name from the slight delay from the time of depolarization to the time of actually opening. The evidence indicates these potassium channels are opening at progressively depolarizing voltages. This is a very unique property of the potassium channels as it is important in the manner of repolarization in some neurons. This time delay is an important function of the depolarization and repolarization of the neuron. Another subtype of potassium channels are those that are activated by Ca^{2+}. In this channel subtype, the inactivation of the channel is the function. It requires the concentration of the intracellular Ca^{2+} to be available in conjunction with the K^{+}. There is a class of potassium channels, "A Channels" that have properties like the sodium channel, they show rapid increase in the current produced with depolarization but then they have a slow decay of channel activity. These channel subtypes are seen only in prolonged excitability. The prototypic channel of this design is the myocardial cell extended activation mechanism. Other potassium channels are seen to have a voltage gate type of behavior. They are activated while the membrane is more negative and not more positive.

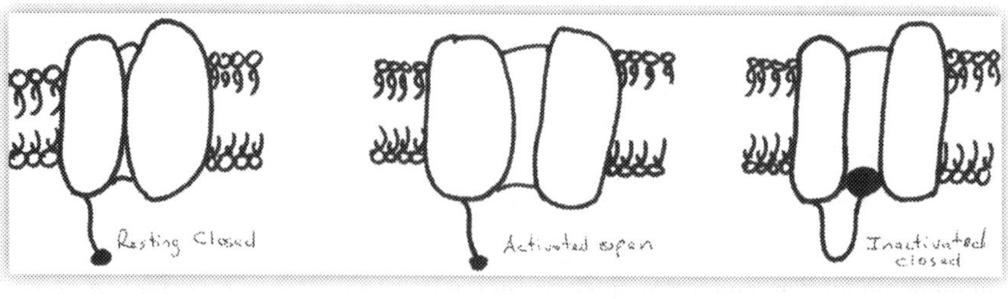

The sodium channel is the best understood of the channels. Especially the voltage gated sodium channel. The sodium channel has been shown to open prior to the K^+ channel is one of the most basic principles of the neuron. The Na^+ channel has a differing behavior. From a structural standpoint, the sodium channel composes close to 1% of the total transmembrane proteins of the neuron. The Na^+ voltage gated channels demonstrated in the diagram show several configurations of the gates. These gates respond to the depolarization of the membrane by activation of the channel. The same depolarization will elicit a move towards the closed state of the channel, with a period of both gates being open at the same time. This unusual configuration of this channel subtype produces a slight time delay between the two channels and produces a situation of three states of the two channels, active, inactive and resting. The activation of the opening of the active channel is very rapid and allows the influx rate of sodium to be in excess of 10^7 ions/sec, where the inactivation is slower. The nature of this active state has the active channel open and the inactive gate open, where the resting state has the activation gate closed and finally the inactive state where the active gate open and the inactive gate closed. The product of all these states will be a transition of the sodium ion flux across the membrane being prolonged and the resultant alteration in membrane potential being prolonged.

In reviewing the activity of the sodium-potassium channels, there is a need to understand the resultant effect of these ions as they flow through the ion channels. We look at the neuron in relation to what it does as a job, transmit information, modulate information and receive information. These functions must be performed in portions of a second. This means that the neuron must have a mechanism to be able to perform these activities in rapid succession. In this type situation, the neuron is not always activated and so we have to have a beginning point of reference. In the neuron we will call this the resting membrane potential or (Vm). In practical application, this is a very minute period of time in relative time of existence. This process of remaining at rest is an energy expensive process. This is due to the continual disruption of the soma by many EPSP's and IPSP's that bombard the neuron cell body. In order for this resting membrane potential to be established there must be the structural lipid bilayer to separate the charges, the ion channels as described to allow the eventual flux of the opposing charged ions and some mechanism of pushing these ions in or out of the cell. The neuron uses a pump to move the ions in or out as required in addition to the simple gradient of charge movement associated with the opposing charges. In our analogy of the electric circuit, the lipid bilayer becomes the capacitor, being relative unaffected by the charge of the ions surrounding it. It is described as being impermeable to the ions within the cell as well as those outside the cell. This property of impermeability is what makes it analogous to the dielectric component.

In the simple circuit, there is a battery (power source) and a resistor. In this scenario, the power source is where the voltage is produced. The voltage value represented will exhibit a reduction as it travels across the circuit. This is the voltage difference (V) that is measured as the ions travel along the circuit and through the resistor. The voltage from the source will cause a movement of the ions across the circuit that is called the current (I). This is the same if we discuss the wiring of a house or a movement of ions in a solution in the laboratory. The movement of the ions in the circuit will move from the negative pole of the voltage source or batter towards the positive pole of the source or battery. The reverse situation is true for the movement of the ions through the circuit, they will move from the positive pole towards the negative through the resistor. In terms of the circuit, it is called a closed circuit. The mathematical expression of this flow of ions can be defined by Ohm's Law. The battery is the portion of this closed circuit that produces the voltage source. In cellular terms the battery is analogous to the ion potential difference. This in turn will produce the potential difference across the cell membrane. The voltage (V) will in turn create a drive of ions through the circuit against a resistance. This movement of ions is termed the current (I). It can be expressed as Ohm's Law $V=IR$. V is the ion potential difference across the cell membrane, the resistor (R) and this value is expressed in volts (V). The resistance is the ability of the cell membrane to impede the flow of the current. In this equation, I is expressed in terms of amperes (A). Thus, conductance is the inverse of the resistance such that conductance (G) is expressed as $G = I/R$. A good conductor is a material that has very little resistance while a good insulator is a material that has a very high resistance. In the case of the nervous system, the conductance is expressed in terms of seimens (S).

In the model described above, there is no net transfer or separation of the charge across the resistor. In order to mimic the human nervous system, we must introduce the idea of charge separation, so we must introduce the capacitor to the system. It is the capacitor that allows for the charged ions to accumulate and create an equal but opposite accumulation of the opposite charged ions on the other side of the capacitor, thus creating a separation of charge. The capacitor will store some value of charge and this is calculated by the formula Q=CV where Q is the amount of charge within the capacitor (coulombs) and the capacitance is expressed as farads (F) and the voltage (V).

The internal milieu consists of differing ionic concentrations that are separated by a lipid bilayer called the plasma membrane or the cell membrane. This structural feature was discussed above and again demonstrates its significance as the discussion of this resting membrane potential begins to show a larger overview of the process. In order for the charge of the cell to change it electrical charge, there must be a net flux of these charged ions through the cell membrane. For these changes to occur, the membrane must allow a flow of charged particles across its lipid bilayer or insulator. The electrical potential that each cell exhibits in its "natural "state is called it's resting membrane potential (Vm).

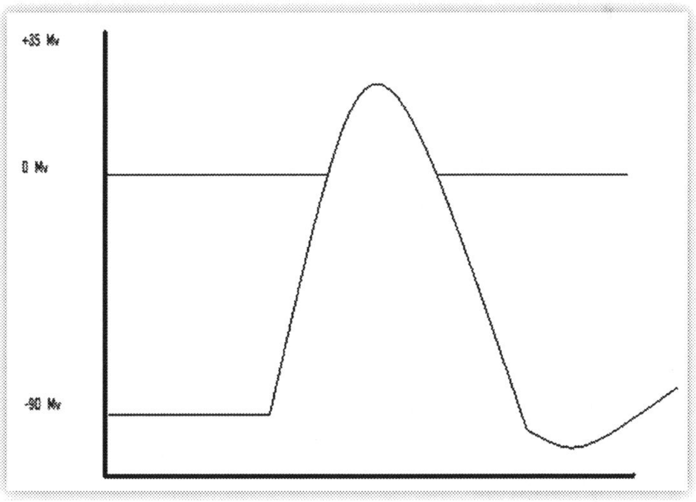

Time

The maintenance of this potential is kept via membrane structure (lipid bilayer) membrane channels (gated), membrane permeability, molecular size and ionic charge. The lipid bilayer produces the separation of the internal ions and those found outside the cell in the extracellular fluid. It is the passage of the ions through the membrane via these channels or pores that generate the current, defined as the ions/second. It is important to remember that the electrical resistance of the neuron is inversely proportional to the number of ion channels present in the membrane and the conductance of the neuron to a specific ion is proportional to the permeability of the membrane to that ion. The pores of a membrane are formed from protein complexes. These protein complexes are arranged to make channels for the exclusive purpose of transporting ions through and exclusion of ions, as discussed above. The channels are ion specific, specific for size, specific for shell of hydration, etc. In the human nervous system, the resting nerve membrane is semi-permeable to Cl- and K+ while at the same time being impermeable to Na+. Regulation of the relative concentration of these ions is due to the diffusion potential of each ion. If the same number of ions are diffused in as those diffused out then the cell ionic potential is at zero. So in electric terms, the ionic gradient is the battery, the voltage being the equilibrium potential and the resistance being the internal milieu of the cell and the conductivity being the membrane of the cell and its permeability. Ions are able to move across the membrane in a passive nature because of the electrochemical force generated by the concentrations of each ion. Mathematically, this is expressed as the Nernst potential. This equation is important as the membrane potential is influenced the most by the concentration changes in the ion that has the greatest flux, and the membrane potential that approximates the Nernst potential of the ion with the greatest flux.

In the human nervous system, the electric potential is called the electrochemical gradient. Thus, the polarity of the cell is determined by the net flux of the charged ions. In the cell the charged ions that are important in this regulation are the intracellular Cl- and Na+ and the extracellular K+. The resting membrane potential is maintained by membrane pumps. These pumps are responsible for pumping three Na+ molecules out of the cell for every two K+ it pumps in. These pumps require ATP for the energy needed to pump ions in and out of the cell. The numbers of ions pumped in and out are not equal therefore a slight depolarization of the cell is seen due to the two K+ pumped in and the three Na+ pumped out. It is important to note that Cl- is not actively pumped but it does contribute to the potential charge across the membrane. Given this property, the energy requirement for the pump must be accounted for during the metabolic requirements of the system.

Extacellular vs. Intracellular ion concentration

IONS	EXTRACELLULAR CONCENTRATION	INTRACELLULAR CONCENTRATION
Na+	120mM/L	12mM/L
K+	5mM/L	130mM/L
Cl^-	125mM/L	5mM/L
Ca^{2+}	2mM/L	0.0001mM/L

The ion channel as was discussed earlier is unique in its structure. The ion channel is designed in such a manner that it will assist in the coordination of the flux of ions through the channel. There are regions of the channel that are thought to be "coordination sites" for the ions on the journey through the channel. The coordination sites are thought to direct the positioning of the ion and its ability to expend very little energy on this trip through the cell membrane. The main event in this flux of the ions across the cell membrane is the conformational change of the membrane channel itself. The conformational change is in fact an alteration of the actual structure of the transmembrane protein. The changes are structural in nature and are responsible for the "open "and the "closed" positions. This conformational change must be induced by a specific mechanism. It has been experimentally demonstrated that the channels will altered by the change in voltage or the binding of a ligand. Ligand channels are seen most often in the second messenger systems that will be discussed later in this book. It is these two properties that have given rise to the naming of the channels as either a ligand gated channel or a voltage gated channel. The voltage gated channel is found to be imperative in the shaping of the action potential and the initiation of the action potential as well. In the major portion of the channel that is voltage gated, the channel is named for the ion that the channel is selective for. The ligand gated channel is specific for a specific ligand. The actual receptor site on the ligand gated channel is the site of the specificity. The best understood of this channel type is the nicotinic acetylcholine receptor in the neuromuscular junction of skeletal muscle. This is considered the "gold standard" of the ligand gated channels. The twist in these two channel descriptions is in the appearance of the channel that is responsive to both stimuli. In this instance the channel is responsive to the binding of the specific ligand but the ligand binding will actually create a voltage change in the membrane as the ion passes through the channel. There are some channels that are able to alter the conformational structure through the binding of a distant receptor. In this instance the ligand will bind to a distant molecule and through the binding elicit a cascade of molecular interactions that will induce the conformational change. The binding of second messengers are examples of this type of channel.

As was previously mentioned, the ion channel is able to discern specific ions as they attempt to penetrate the membrane. The channel itself has structural aspects that allow for this ionic selectivity. These channels are selective on the basis of the ion sign at the very least. By the charge being positive or negative is the most fundamental aspect of discrimination available for the channel. Selectivity is also based on the molecular size of the ion. The experimental evidence on the sodium channel allowing for the free passage of the sodium ion and then limiting the passage of the potassium ion has been demonstrated and supports this selectivity method. The data has been so well studied and demonstrated that a review of this process is not warranted. The confirmation of the theory is seen in the reverse situation, where the potassium channel will allow for the free passage of the much larger potassium ion, but limits the passage of the much smaller sodium ion. Additional selectivity is possible through the structural architecture of the channel. By the size of the hydrophobic pocket, the selectivity of the channel is again regulated. The membrane of the cell will respond to the alterations in the internal charge difference by either increasing or decreasing the permeability to the cell.

The actual opening of the channel is termed a pore. This pore is the hollow opening of the transmembrane protein allowing the passage of the ions through the membrane. Action potentials of the vast majority of nerve cells is derived from the voltage gated Na^+ and K^+ channels. Even as the two channels are responsible for a like end result, the channels are vastly different. The potassium channel is a very simplistic channel with only a single gate. The gate only has a single activating component, that of depolarization. As the cell depolarizes, the channel moves to the open configuration or activated state. This conformation is responsible for the regulation of the potassium ions traversing the membrane. The sodium channel is much more complex in structure as compared to the potassium channel. The sodium channel has experimentally been found to possess two differing conformations. This corresponds to the two voltage sensitive gates of the sodium channel. The two gates are made of the activation gate and the inactivation gate. The activation gate is analogous to the activation gate of the potassium channel in the depolarization of the cell is responsible for the opening of the gate. The inactivation gate is not like the potassium gate since the depolarization of the cell will move the gate into the closed conformation. At a glance opposite actions of the two gates would lead one to believe that the activity of the two gates will cancel each other out. This is not the fact of the function of the gate. Built into the sodium channel is a delay in the opening of the activation with depolarization and the closing of the inactivation gate. With depolarization, there will be a period of both gates being open, with the inactivation gates beginning to close first. The structure of the sodium channel allows for three stages of the channel conformational structure, resting where the activation gate is closed and the inactivation gate is open, activated configuration where both channels are open, and finally, the inactivated configuration where the activation gate is open and the inactivation gate is closed. These conformational states are the functional characteristics of the action potential.

In the function of the nerve cell, dissipation of the ion gradient would mean total loss of charge difference and therefore loss of neurological function. It has been well understood that the diffusional abilities of ions are not strong enough to maintain the electrochemical gradient that is required for the membrane potential discussed above. Therefore, there must be another mechanism available to maintain the gradient differences. The structures that tare able to ensure that the electrochemical differences are maintained in the extracellular compartment versus the intracellular environment are the ion pumps. Much research has been done on the functional and structural role of these pumps. It is not the intention of this discussion to delve deeply into this subject at this point but mention must be made as to the mechanism of action as to how the pumps work. In order for the electrochemical gradient to be maintained there must be a flow of ions against the concentration gradient. This movement of ions against the concentration gradient requires energy. In solution, the electrochemical potential of the ion is proportional to the concentration of that ion in the solution. The laws of physics will have the movement of these ions in such a manner that they will try to reduce the potential energy of the gradient from areas of greater concentration to areas of lower concentrations. This solidifies the requirement for the input of energy to move against this potential energy. In the nervous system, the energy that is supplied to perform this work is in the form of Adenosine Triphosphate or ATP. The molecules of ATP will be hydrolyzed to provide the energy required to move ions against the electrochemical gradients. The best studied ion pump in the nervous system is the sodium-potassium pump that shuttles sodium ions and potassium ions between the extracellular environments to the intracellular environment. The sodium ions will interact with the receptor sites on the cytoplasmic aspect of the pump while the potassium ions will bind to the extracellular aspect of the transmembrane protein. The binding will cause a conformational change as mentioned previously, and the transfer of the ions will be that there will be a gain of potassium ions into the cell and the sodium ions lost to the extracellular environment. This pumping action is the basis of the electrochemical gradient that is seen in the nervous system. In this particular pump, the accounting of the ions is not a straight one to one relationship. In this particular ion pump, there is a situation where there will be a net flux of three sodium ions for two potassium ions. It is believed that this discrepancy of ions transfer is in part responsible for the voltage associated with the resting membrane potential.

The ion pumps and the ion channels are both able to translocate across the cell membrane of a nerve cell. The channels and the pumps are highly selective in the ions they allow passage through the cell membrane. Why then would a molecule look to a channel versus a pump? In the structural considerations of the ion channel, the constraints are such that passage of the ions through the transmembrane protein channel is much faster then that for the pump. The numbers of sodium ions that are able to pass though the sodium channel in a single second have been measured to be greater than ten million ions. This is in stark contrast to the numbers associated with the sodium-potassium pump. In the pump the numbers have been demonstrated to be as few as one thousand ions per second. Additionally, there is consideration of the effects of temperature on the neural cell membrane. As the cell membrane increases temperature there is seen to be a concurrent increase in the transport of the ions across the cell membrane. This structural characteristic would explain the concern associated with pathologic increases in body core temperature and or pH.

In addition to the structural aspect of the ion channel the genetic encoding that is seen with each type of channel will play a part in the channel behavior. The genetic encoding of very specific amino acid sequences plays an important role in the functional regulation of the passage of ions through the cell membrane. The ability of genetic studies to look into the primary sequencing of these gene signals has revealed some common aspect in these encoding regions. These commonalities are demonstrated from a variety of organisms and not solely in humans. It is due to this ability of genetic studies to identify the common aspects of these genes from organism to organism, that has led to several of the genes being called "superfamilies of genes".

CHAPTER 7

ELECTROCHEMICAL POTENTIAL

The human nervous system is continually being bombarded with inputs from the external environment as well as the internal environment. The numbers of these inputs make the functional accuracy of the system even more amazing as a better understanding of this mechanism is obtained. In addition to the inputs, there is modulation and integration of the signaling that is the function of the nervous system as well as interpretation of the data. In the capacity of the brain and the nervous system as the intelligence of the human, there is a tremendous amount of activity for even the most simple of activities, let alone the most complex activities. The idea of thought processing, integration into learning of motor behaviors as well as memory traces shows the complexity of the system and all that it is required to do. In the previous chapter, the principle of the ion channel was discussed. This chapter will look into the result of the activity of the ion channel. We understand the potential difference across the lipid bilayer due to the separation of charge. It is the basic tenant of the whole system of operation. In the human nervous system, the interior of the cell is kept more negative than the exterior of the cell. Experimentally, we have demonstrated this potential difference to be measured at between -40mV to -90mV (millivolts). The neuron and the system are dependent upon the exchange of the ions and the flux to stimulate the neuron. In the situation where the value internally becomes less negative, it is depolarized, and excited. The reverse is that the cell moves more to a more negative value within the cell and becomes hyperpolarized or inhibited. In the previous chapter, the structure of the channel was discussed and here the theories of activation and inactivation will be discussed. The lipid bilayer provides an exceptional insulation to prevent the inadvertent flux of ions. It is a structure that is incredibly well designed for this job, being thin and yet fluid and strong. It allows the flux of ions in and out of the cell via gated pores. This regulation of the charge is done through the regulation of the flow of ions across the membrane. The ability to regulate this flow is via two interrelated mechanisms, the gating of the channel and the ion selectivity of the channel. These pores allow the selective movement of the ions based on charge, size and electrochemical gradient. Ion channels that are selective for a positive charged monovalent cation such as Na^{+}, K^{+} will not allow the flow of negatively charged anions through the channel, the Cl^{-} or sulfates. The ability to transition between the active or "open" state to the inactive or "closed" state is the process defined as "gating". In the closed state it is assumed that there is little to no flow of ions through that specific channel.

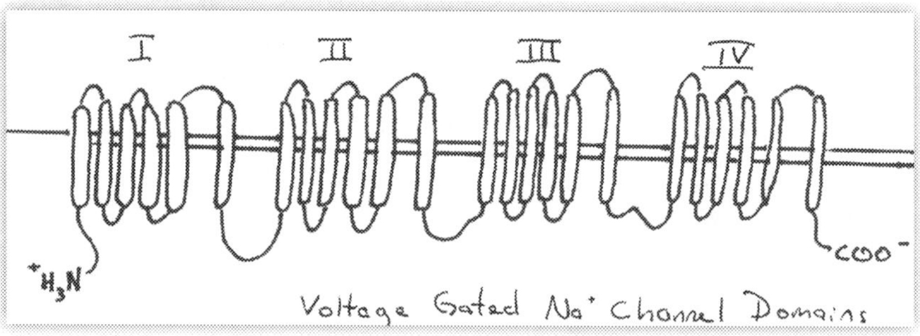

It is important to remember that in the neuron, the current is reflective of the flux of the ions as they move through the membrane as compared to time. In the majority of the channels presented in this text, there will be a conformational change in the channel as it transitions from the open or "active" state and the closed or "inactive" state. The movement of the ion is a phenomenon that can be calculated mathematically by the Nernst

Potential. It is a formula that will describe the ion concentration as it is related to the generation of electrical potential.

Nernst formula:

$$Ex = \frac{RT}{zF} \ ln \frac{[X]o}{[X]i}$$

R = gas constant

T= temp in degrees Kelvin

z = valence of the ion

F= faraday constant (charge of 1 mole of monovalent ion)

X_o = extracellular ion concentration

X_i = intracellular ion concentration

The units of the response will be in volts.

The Nernst formula will predict the specific value of the membrane potential under whatever limiting variable presents that the membrane is selectively and exclusively permeable to that sole ion. This theory is our basis of the functional capacity of the human nervous system.

The gating that is described by the mathematical representation is a function of the change in the shape or the configuration of the channel and its cytoarchitecture. These changes in conformation will be made possible due to the stimuli presented to the neuron channel, voltage or ligand binding. Many of the channels in the nervous system are voltage gated in nature and others are affected by the binding of a ligand. The voltage gated ion channel is influenced by the alteration of the membrane potential (Vm). These channels are involved with the initiation and the conduction of the impulses that the neuron will transmit. The vast majority of the ion channels are named for the ion that they are influenced by, such as the Na^+, K^+, Cl^-, Ca^+, etc. The ligand gated channels are influenced by the binding of the ligand. There must be a binding of a specific ligand to the specific receptor as has been previously discussed. The binding of this ligand will initiate a variety of responses. The most well investigated of this class is the neuromuscular junction in which the nicotinic ACh receptor of skeletal muscle is the receptor for the ACh ligand. There is a third class of channel in which there is a dual activation of the channel. The channel will respond to both the voltage differential and the binding of the ligand. The Ca^{+} - K^{+} channel is prototypic of this classification dual activation channel. The other channel well investigated is the dopamine—K^{+} channel where the binding of the dopamine will activate a membrane bound GTP protein that will in turn elicit the opening of the K^{+} channel.

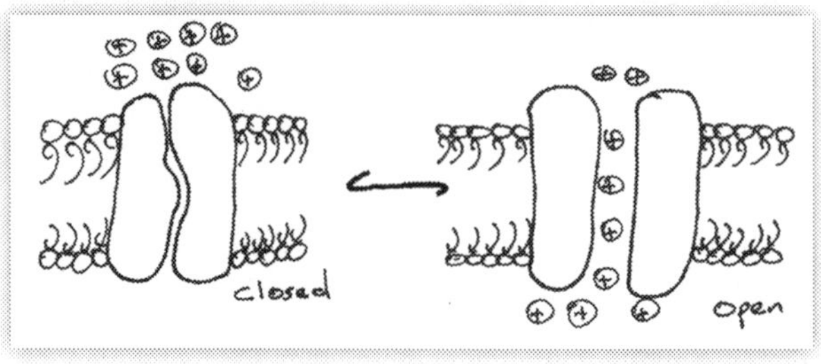

It has been well documented that the selective permeability based on ion charge, or ligand or duality incorporates a subclassification of size if molecule. The idea that the size is important was demonstrated with the investigation of the rationale of the 50-100 times greater permeability to K^{+} ions in the potassium channel to the smaller Na^{+} ion. It is believed that the mechanism of action in this selectivity may be the alteration in the amino acid sequencing of the channel pore. The calcium channel is unique in itself as it contains several subtypes. The role of the calcium ion is to improve the release of the neurotransmitter from the cell to stimulation of the activity of a variety of enzymatic activities within the cell. The calcium channels are divided into the L type, the P type and the N type. The location of the L type Ca^{+} channel is found within the majority of muscle tissues. This includes the skeletal, cardiac and smooth muscles. What is important to the neuroscientist and the neurologist is the understanding that there are L type channels found within the neuronal cell body. This type of channel is designed to assist in the depolarization process of the neuron. The N type channel is almost exclusively found within the neuron. They function in the importation of calcium into the neuron. There is also evidence that this channel will assist in the release.

The ability to have and to maintain the electrical charge difference between the inside and the outside of the cell is based on the lipid bilayer described in previous chapters. (Chapter 5) In this model of the human nervous system, the inside of the cell is negatively charged with respect to the extracellular space. As mentioned in pervious chapters, the difference in this charge is called the membrane potential, more specifically, the resting membrane potential as the cell is not actively engaged in communication of other function. This value is a slightly variable value but the general accepted range is -70mV to -90mV. Stimulation of the neuron will produce a cascade of events that will lead to alteration of this electrochemical potential difference between the inside of the cell and the external environment. This is due in part to the voltage sensitive ion channels within the membrane of the neuron. The Nernst equation is the mathematical expression of each of the ions variation of this membrane potential as they move across the lipid bilayer. The eventual outcome is an effect on the post synaptic cell membrane or the effector membrane. This mechanism is either going to be an excitatory post synaptic potential (EPSP) or an inhibitory post synaptic potential (IPSP) based upon the neurotransmitter and the receptor involved. When the concentration of an ion on one side of the semipermeable membrane is greater than the concentration on the other side, an electrical potential and therefore a chemical concentration gradient exists. In the resting state, the neuron has a definitive permeability to the three ions (K+, Cl-, Na^+) and the basis for the resting potential (E_M). Alteration of any of the three of these ions will alter the E_M. There is a formula that is utilized to define the parameters of the function of the individual gradient and the permeability (P) of the ion as it relates to the membrane, the Goldman-Hodgkin-Katz equation:

Nernst equation

$$E_K = \frac{RT}{zF} \ln \frac{[K]_o}{[K]_i}$$

Goldman - Hodgkin - Katz equation

$$E_m = \frac{RT}{zF} \ln \frac{P_K[K]_o + P_{Na}[Na]_o + P_{Cl}[Cl]_i}{P_K[K]_i + P_{Na}[Na]_i + P_{Cl}[Cl]_o}$$

The Goldman-Hodgkins-Katz formula is used to predict the behavior of the E_M if the permeability of one ion changes in such a nature that it becomes greater than the others. It clearly demonstrates that the E_M will move in the direction of the Nernst potential for that ion with the concentration change. To understand the membrane potential, the assumption will be made the neuron is in a state of "rest". This indicates a distribution of ions that is unequal across the membrane.

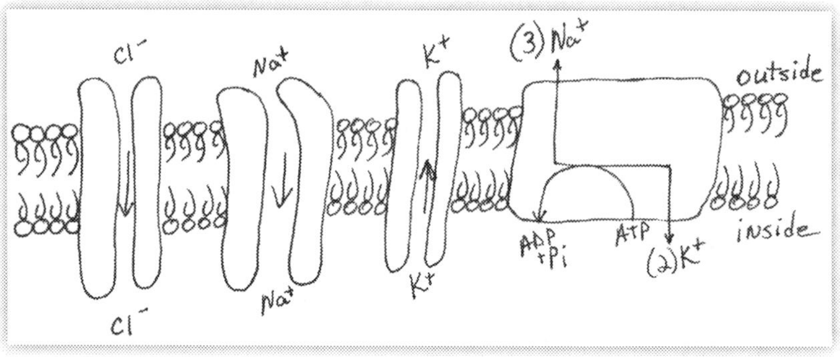

The cell membrane in this example is going to be permeable only to K^+ and thus the P_{Na} and the P_{Cl} will equal 0 and this will indicate that the Goldman-Hodgkins-Katz formula will now represent the Nernst equation for K^+, owing to the formula $E_M = E_{K+}$ =-90mV. Now as we investigate the process let us assume that there is an additional Na^+ channel within the membrane. This indicates that there is an additional amount of charged ion to account for, the new ion is the Na^+ ion and this creates a flow of sodium ions into the cell. The reason for the flow of the Na^+ ions into the cell is due to the 15mM gradient inside the cell and the 140mM gradient outside the cell and thus a concentration gradient drive of ions into the cell. This is in direct conflict with the concentration gradient of K^+ as well, but the chemical repulsion is greater and thus the push of K^+ out of the cell is the result of this chemical concentration gradient. In this situation, the E_M is such that it makes the membrane more permeable to the K^+ ion, with the 4.7 mM outside the cell and the 140mM inside the cell driving this gradient. It is this movement of the ions due to the concentration gradient difference that must be overcome for the efflux of K^+ ions from the cell. The movement of the K^+ ion is the mechanism that the cell uses to negate the effects of the incoming Na^+ ions that are trying to change the E_M. This alteration in the flow of ions as well as the charge moving between the Nernst potential for either of the Na+ or the K^+ ion will create the new E_M that will fall between -90mV and +60mV or close to -75mV. Using this model, it is easy to understand the ease with which the E_M can ne perturbed. It is also easy to understand the complexity of the mechanism that is responsible for the establishment and the maintenance of the E_M. It is important to remember the imbalance of the normal flux of the Na^+ and the K^+ ions as the cell will allow for the removal of (3) Na^+ ions for every (2) K^+ ions. (Na^+ ions out and K^+ ions in) The third ion that is involved in the E_M is the chloride ion. The membrane of the neuron is very permeable to Cl-. This flux of the K+ and the Na^+ ions will dictate the passive flow of the Cl- ion. The manner that the internal aspect of the concentration gradient lies in relation to the Nernst potential for Cl- will dictate the flux of Cl- either to flow in or out of the cell. In the cell—soma synaptic communication calcium is more important for the potentiation of the action potential. This is not true for the movements of Ca^{2+} and Mg^{2+}. These ions are more closely related to Na^+ and K^+ in functional characteristics. These ions are not responsible to any extent that is significant to the contribution of the E_M.

The mechanism of this resting membrane potential and the resultant activity can be looked at through the activity of the voltage sensitive ion channel within the neuron cell membrane. This is because the voltage sensitive Na^+ and K^+ channels are the manner that the neuron utilizes to generate the action potential that is the backbone of how we as humans function. The action potential is the result of the disturbance of the resting membrane potential (E_M). The E_M of the axon is increased from the -75mV position to the more positive +15mV level for a very short but intense period of 4 msec. After this time at the more positive value, the E_M is returned to the normal value of -75mV. In this model, the ability to have the alteration in the E_M, described, there must be a flux of these ions across the membrane. In order for this to take place, there must be a mechanism available for this flow and this is done via the voltage sensitive ion channel. The Na^+ conductance is seen to increase immediately with the channel altering its configuration from the closed state into the open or activated state. It remains in the "open" or "activated "state for milliseconds and then returns to the "inactive state."

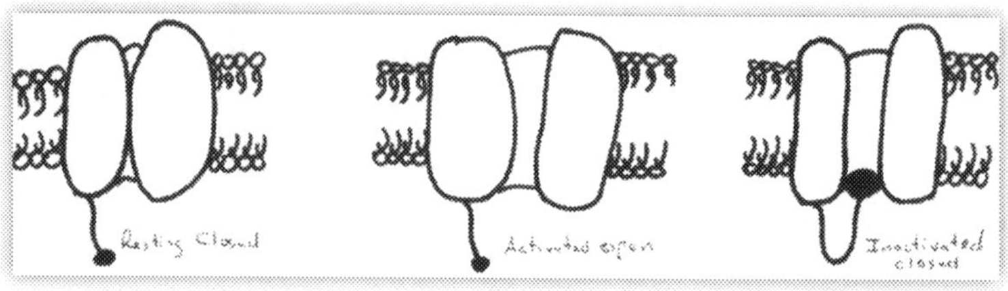

The voltage sensitive Na^+ channels have a unique distribution within the cytoarchitectural make-up of the cell. The concentration of these channels is of primary importance for the specific function of the neuron. These channels are found with a greater distribution at the initial segment of the axon as was discussed in previous chapters. This distribution of channels is on the order of seven (7) times greater in the initial segment than that of the cell body or the dendrite. The depolarization that has spread into the region of increased Na^+ channels, there will be an activation of the Na^+ channels that increases 6,000-7,000 times the conductance of the ions. This rapid proliferation will produce an action potential secondary to the rapid influx of the Na^+ ions into the cell, and thus inwardly directed sodium current. This inward rush of Na^+ ions will then generate the depolarization of the membrane along the anatomic structure called the "initial segment a t the junction of the some and the axon. This structure will then allow for the spread of the electrical alteration into the lateral aspect of the initial segment and produce the charge change in the intracellular fluid based upon that Na^{+-} K+ pump. This sequence of ion flux and resultant charge alteration is then propagated along the axon as what we now describe as an "action potential". In order for this propagated electrical potential to change the membrane potential from the resting state (-75 mV) to a threshold stimulus, there must be a concentration of sodium channels to continue this electrical charge to continue to be altered. From a structural standpoint, the sodium channels are very unique in how they allow for the rapid flow of ions through the channel to create this alteration in membrane potential. They become open or activated and within milliseconds, they will reverse that opening and rapidly move into a closed position. During this point there is a subset of time where both the Na^+ and the K^+ channels are both in the open position or the activated position. This timeframe is a millisecond but it is nonetheless apparent. This transfer of ions is the basis for the return to resting membrane potentials within the cell. Remembering that the opening-closing or the activation-inactivation of these two channels is the defining mechanism of the action potential, it is important to remember that the rapid depolarization of the membrane is due to the sodium channel moving into the open or the active position and the concurrent activation of the potassium channels. It is imperative to understand that the potassium channel responds slower than the sodium channel and as such transfer of K^+ ions is maximal during the repolarization or after potential, reaching the greatest action during the hypolarization phase.

The K^+ channel is different in the manner it responds to the depolarization of the cell, it will be much slower in the response to the depolarization but also more prolonged in the return to the inactive state, creating a more lengthy response to the depolarization. The entire time that the membrane remains depolarized, the K^+ ion channel will remain active. Upon restoration of the E_M, the K^+ channels will then return to the closed state. Therefore, it can be said that the depolarization of the cell is due to the extremely rapid alteration between the two states of the sodium channel and that the return to the repolarized state being due to the voltage sensitive K^+ channel. In the action potential, the peak of the upstroke (flux of Na^+) will elicit a reversal of the potential that will be reflected by the change in ion permeability and thus drive the membrane potential from being closer to the permeability of Na^+ to that of the permeability of K^+. Included in this equation must be the activity of calcium channels, especially when the synaptic activity is directed to the soma. In the course of the reversal of the membrane permeability, the continued opening of the K^+ gated voltage channels will produce a flux of ions back to E_M. This alteration in membrane potential is apparent even with the membrane potential still being more positive (a condition that favors the open state of the Na^+ channel). Associated with this reversal of membrane potential and the open K^+ channels will make K^+ flux dominant. This will allow for the movement of the membrane potential to move to a more negative value. The delay of the K^+ channels will eventually close and the resting membrane potential will be reestablished.

The model that has been discussed throughout this chapter has been that of the neuromuscular junction. In the human nervous system, the spacing between the pre synaptic and the post-synaptic cell is around 20nm. This is the space that is called the synaptic cleft. Within this space there are a number of important chemical actions that will take place. This spacing is also of enough of a distance to prevent the backflow of neurotransmitter. In the scenario that we have discussed, there is an additional ion that must be accounted for and that is calcium. The Ca^+ ion is important in the regulation of the release and uptake of the neurotransmitter at the synaptic terminal. Common behavior to all chemical synapses will be the manner that the activity of the synapse can be described. The chemical activity can be described as the presynaptic activity: release, and then the postsynaptic activity: effect. As has been described previously, the activity within the presynaptic cell will elicit the release of the neurotransmitter substance in amounts that are defined as quanta.

CHAPTER 8

BIOCHEMISTRY OF NEUROTRANSMISSION

Neurotransmitters are the basis of every aspect of the human brain that we are able to imagine. Every thought, action, behavior, movement, memory and perception is made possible by the biochemical processes of a neurotransmitter. There are many theories of how these substances exist and act. In ancient Chinese theology, the predominant theory was that a substance called chi flowed in channels within the body. It was the basis for the workings of acupuncture called tai chi. Before this description was that of the Greeks and the Romans. The Greek physicians and the Roman physicians describe a substance called pneuma. This substance was believed to be produced in the lungs and the heart. These theories were the basis of further investigations.

There are specific criteria that must be met for a substance to be considered as a neurotransmitter.

1. The substance must be present in appropriate amounts in the presynaptic process.

2. Enzymes that synthesize the substance must be present and active in the presynaptic terminal. The enzymes that degrade it must also be present in the synaptic space.
3. Stimulation of the presynaptic axon should cause release of the substance while application of an analogue should elicit like effect on the nerve.
4. Drugs that effect specific enzymatic or receptor-mediated effects of the proposed neurotransmitter should also alter the nerve stimulation through changes in the synthesis, storage, release, uptake or stimulation or blockage of the receptor.

Neurotransmitter can be biogenic amines like the catecholamines norepinepherine and dopamine and the indolamines serotonin and histamine. Neurotransmitters can also be acetylcholine, amino acids or small proteins. Amino acids that are used as neurotransmitters are Gamma-Aminobutyric acid (GABA), glycine or glutamate. If the substance is a neuropeptide it is most often synthesized in the cell body and then transported to the axon via axonal transport. Neurotransmitter can be either excitatory or inhibitatory in their effect.

Another type of transmitter is called the Neurohormone. Neurohormones are chemical messengers that are secreted by the brain into the circulatory system that elicit their effect by altering the cellular functions. These are referred to as peptide neurohormones if they are synthesized and secreted from the hypothalamus. These neurohormones are secreted directly into the portal circulation and from there carried to the Anterior Pituitary. It is here in the anterior pituitary that they exert the effect upon the endocrine system. Neurohormones are powerful effectors within the spinal cord and brainstem. They also have effects upon a variety of other areas of the brain as well. It is possible, if not definitive that there is a coexistence of a cofactor for certain neurotransmitters. It is conceivable that the cofactor or co-transmitter can be released from the same nerve terminal. The co-transmitters are modulators and function in the role of being a modulator. [Fig 1]

NEUROTRANSMITTER	COTRANSMITTER
Catecholamines Dopamine Norepinepherine Epinephrine	CCK, enkephalin Neuropeptide Y, Neurotensin, enkephalin Enkephalin, Neuropeptide Y
Serotonin	CCK, enkephalin, Substance P
Acetylcholine	VIP, Substance P, Enkephalin, CGRP
GABA	Enkephalin, Neuropeptide Y, CCK
Glutamate	Substance P
Glycine	Neurotensin

In this role they are called autocoids. It is also possible that the neurotransmitter itself acts as a modulator. Evidence of this is seen in the peripheral nervous system where norepinepherine in the post synaptic receptor can be excitatory in its effect on the post synaptic receptor and concurrently stimulate a presynaptic receptor as an inhibitor to prevent further release of norepinepherine. The actual tissue involved in this instance is in the heart as a post synaptic tissue and the alpha 2 as a presynaptic tissue

Classical neurotransmitters are small (30 nm in diameter) and are stored in the synaptic vesicles that are produced in the axon terminal itself. It is the larger co-transmitters that are synthesized in the neuronal cell body, or the soma itself and then transported to the axon using axonal transport. The smaller transmitter vesicles are highly concentrated within the active zone of the terminal. The active zone will be visualized as an area of electron dense regions where there are increased numbers of calcium channels. There is a tremendous amount of mitochondrial activity see in these regions as well due to the tremendous amount of energy requirements needed for the production of the synaptic vesicles. The calcium channels are a low frequency channel and as such are stimulated will cause a large alteration in the permeability of the cell membrane with regards to calcium.

Calcium ions rush in and this initiates the cascade of the release of the neurotransmitter via the synaptic vesicles.

The synaptic vesicle will stain intensely for the suspected neurotransmitter with histological technique. The vesicle with the neurotransmitter will fuse with the cell membrane and by a process of exocytosis release its contents to the synaptic cleft or space. The amount of the neurotransmitter released is called quanta. The vesicle will then be re-used many times by the axon terminal for this process. The co-transmitters are larger peptides and are found in the larger vesicles in separate areas of the axon distant to the active zone.

The frequency required for the release of the smaller vesicles is a lower frequency than that required to liberate the larger vesicles. Since in some instances, the co-transmitter and the neurotransmitter itself are released from the same terminal there can be experimental models designed to identify these dual role axon terminals.

Transmitters can be classified as either fast or slow. This classification is dependent upon the whether the effect are long lasting or short acting. These effects are able to range from milliseconds to hours to days even. Acetylcholine and the amino acids acting at the nicotinic receptors because rapid postsynaptic affects that are measured in milliseconds. This is possible due to the ion channels found within the nerve membrane. Acetylcholine and glutamate receptors are composed of 5 protein subunits that compromise the ion channel for calcium and sodium. Again, the structure of the receptor allows for millisecond response times. Conversely, acetylcholine at the muscarinic receptor as well as the catecholamines induces a slow change in the target tissue that can last for several seconds to minutes. The mechanism here is a single subunit protein channel that is coupled to a G protein. The fast transmitters act via a change in the distribution of the ion flow through the specific channel that causes a change of the electrical potential and thus a change in the biochemistry within the cell. The changes may include phosphorylation of specific proteins, activation of certain enzymes, and activation of a second messenger system and even activation of translation of increased protein production by increasing genetic translation activity.

Small molecular weight transmitters are synthesized locally within the nerve cell axon or the dendrite itself. The most well understood of the small molecular weight transmitters and modulators are the three amino acid and the five biogenic amines (decarboxylate derivatives of amino acids) and acetylcholine. Each of these are synthesized in the cell body and then transported to the terminal by axonal transport. It is within the axon itself where the synthesis of the neurotransmitter actually occurs.

Acetylcholine is considered to be the prototype neurotransmitter. It is the first to be isolated and thus studied. The nerve systems that utilize acetylcholine are considered cholinergic nerves. These cholinergic nerves are found in the peripheral nervous system, with limited amounts within the central nervous system. In the peripheral nervous system, the pathways that use the cholinergic system will include motor pathways that have origin within the ventral root of the spinal cord. These pathways will innervate the striated skeletal muscle, the preganglionic sympathetic and parasympathetic nerves originating in the mediolateral column of the spinal cord and the brain stem. Postganglionic parasympathetic nerves to the heart, pulmonary bronchi, GI, bladder, eye, exocrine glands are also included in the cholinergic path of nerves. Post ganglionic sympathetic nerves to the major sweat glands are also included within this category. Differences in the nervous system are seen in the Post synaptic receptors that will act on the target tissue. In the neuromuscular junction and the autonomic ganglia, the receptors respond to the drug nicotine, and are thus called nicotinic. The heart and the lungs respond to a drug called muscarine and as such the receptors are celled muscarinic. The innervation is from the parasympathetic nervous system. Cholinergic nerve receptors are found in the brain in a formal proportion, and the muscarinic receptors are 10-100 fold greater than the nicotinic receptors.

The cholinergic paths are seen throughout the brain and form many differing functions. Examples are in the cholinergic cell bodies of the tegmentum that innervate the hypothalamus and the thalamus, while in the striatum, there is experimental evidence that clearly demonstrates the function of these paths in central motor control. Atropine is utilized to block the tremor associated with Parkinson's disease and defines the path from the striatum as a motor control path. In theories of memory, acetylcholine has been demonstrated to play a role in the consolidation of memory traces. The evidence of this is seen where changes occur in the cholinergic receptors if patients with Alzheimer's disease. A cholinergic axon has the ability to synthesize, store and secrete acetylcholine quite independently from the cell body. In this process, the uptake of choline is the rate limiting step in the reaction. The synthesis of acetylcholine requires choline and acetyl coenzyme A to be taken up in the terminal through the enzyme choline acyltransferase. This enzyme has a molecular weight of about 67,000kd. This enzyme is ribosomally synthesized within the cell body and transported via axonal transport to the axon terminal. This is a cytoplasmic enzyme. It carries a positive charge that makes it associate with the intracellular, mitochondrial or vesicular membrane. It adheres via the negative charge associated with the transmembrane carbohydrates. Choline is a component of the complex lipids of all cell membranes. Given this cellular structural fact, one can extrapolate that the cell must have a pump mechanism to promote the uptake of the Choline into the cell. Experimental evidence shows that not only are there pumps that perform this function but that there are differences with the activity of each subtype. In a non-cholinergic cell, the pumps are of a low affinity (400km-100um) subtype. Acetyl coenzyme A is produced within the nerve terminal itself. The acetylcholine is synthesized and then stored in the electron dense granules along with a small amount of ATP (1 M) and a charged anion called vesiculin.

In order for a substance to be considered as a neurotransmitter, there must be a manner for that substance to be cleared from the synapse. In the case of acetylcholine, the enzyme that performs this task is acetylcholinersterase. By definition, the substance must be cleared from the synapse and in this particular case, the enzyme has two forms. True acetylcholinesterase is associated with the neuromuscular junction and is seen within the synaptic cleft. The second form of acetylcholinesterase is found in various other regions of the brain. The greatest concentration of these substances being those areas of increased density of cholinergic neurons within the brain. Both of the subtypes are fast acting enzymes but the true acetylcholinesterase is considered to be one of the fastest enzymes in the body. The Vmax of this enzyme has been measured at a rate of 75g of substrate per hour with 1 mg of pure enzyme. The Choline formed from the degradation of the acetylcholine is actively pumped back into the cell at the nerve terminal and then reused for synthesis of additional acetylcholine. This requires a high affinity pump (Km 0.4-4.0um) to rapidly pump the Choline that has been produced from the degradation of the acetylcholine in the synaptic cleft back into the cell. This is the rate limiting step in the production of this particular neurotransmitter.

In biochemistry as in other chemistries, there is variability on the naming of compounds. This is true with the naming of biogenic amines that function as neurotransmitters. Those that are synthesized from tyrosine are called catecholamines. This is because of the catechol moiety of a phenol ring and 2 hydroxyls. But they are also referred to as adrenergic because of the English term Adrenaline. Additionally, serotonin or 5 Hydroxytryptamine is referred to as a biogenic amine. There is discrepancy in this naming due to the structure of serotonin having an indolamine ring. The ring arises from the tryptophan within the molecule. Histamine is also a biogenic amine that is located within the brain and the GI tract. This transmitter is the decarboxylated form of the amino acid histamine. This is the same histamine that is found in the mast cell and is responsible for the compliment cascade.

The catecholamine transmitters' norepinepherine, epinephrine and dopamine provide a multitude of functions in both the central and peripheral nervous system. The Adrenal Medulla has the capacity the neurotransmitter and the neurohormone epinephrine. When exposed to a light source, the catecholamines oxidize to a colored substance called quinines. The reaction is the same if exposed to an alkaline pH. It is this characteristic that assisted in the identification of the substantia nigra of the midbrain. It was found that the brain, especially the areas know as the substantia nigra would darken when exposed to air. This is because of the high concentration of dopamine within the substantia nigra. Dopamine exerts effects on the renal blood flow as well to round out the varied effects of these biogenic amines.

Tyrosine is the immediate precursor of all three of the catecholamine transmitters, dopamine, norepinepherine, and epinephrine. T He enzymes responsible for the synthesis of the transmitters are themselves synthesized in the cell body by ribosomal proteins. They are then sent off to the terminal to be modified and utilized at the terminal. Structurally, at the terminal imports the needed tyrosine and phenylalanine for this modification.

The reaction goes like this:

Tyrosine is either converted to L Dopa, dopamine, norepinepherine or epinephrine. The enzymes required for this reaction to take place are tyrosine hydroxylase, l-amino acid hydroxylase, dopamine B-hydroxylase, phenylethanolamine-N-methyltransferase. Tyrosine hydroxylase is the first and the rate limiting step for the synthesis of all three catecholamines. It is found within the cytoplasm and requires molecular oxygen, iron and tetrahydrobiopterin as cofactors. It is the function of the cofactor to maintain the enzyme in its reduced and activated state. If the levels of catecholamines like dopamine or norepinepherine within the cytoplasm increase, they will inhibit the peteridine from activation of the tyrosine hydroxylase. It is the end product inhibition that provides for the rate limiting control of the neurotransmitter synthesis. It is also called a negative feedback loop. Tyrosine hydroxylase can be phosphorylated to increase the affinity of the peteridine cofactor. Cyclic 3'5'AMP is the allosteric activator in the presynaptic terminal receptor that also acts as a regulatory step. Intracellular calcium is another mediator of the synthesis of the neurotransmitters that belong to the catecholamine family. This is a classic example of how a second messenger system works. When tyrosine is hydroxylated by tyrosine hydroxylase, the product is an amino acid L-Dopa (L-3, 4 dihydrooxyphenylalanine). In order to control the synthesis of the end product of this reaction, the intermediate of this reaction is decarboxylated in the cytoplasm by another enzyme, L-amino acid decarboxylase. The enzymes L-amino acid decarboxylase and dopamine B hydroxylase yield and end product rate that is 10 to 1000 times greater than the rate of tyrosine hydroxylase. This activity is dependent on the availability of the cofactors required (pyridol phosphate—B6) for L-amino acid hydroxylase.

Dopamine is a unique neurotransmitter in that it is evidenced as the primary catecholamine in the brain of mammals. It is found within the autonomic ganglia, and concurrently it is a neurohormone in the hypothalamus and it controls pituitary secretion of prolactin. In the dopaminergic neurons, it is found in the secretory granules that are to be released by exocytosis.

In the adrenergic nerves of the brain or in the adrenal medulla, norepinepherine diffuses out of the granules containing dopamine B hydroxylase. It is them converted by phenylethanolamine N Methyltransferase (PNMT) using S-adenosylmethonine to produce epinephrine or adrenaline. This is packed into another vesicle that contains ATP, chromogranin and the catecholamines. The adrenal steroid cortisol is the activation control of the enzyme PNMT. The release and activation of the system of synthesis is a cyclic process as well as a stimulatory byproduct. In the morning there is diurnal increase in the secretion of cortisol that activates the PNMT to enhance the synthesis of epinephrine. The epinephrine in turn increases the liver glycolysis, gluconeogenesis and initiates the body for the beginning of its anticipated activities. Termination of the catecholamine transmission occurs by the active reuptake of the biogenic amines by the nerve terminal itself. This process of recycled substances is the product of the degradation of the acetylcholine by the enzyme acetylcholinesterase. It appears that most cells, including platelets are equipped with pumps to pump the catecholamines across the cell membrane. The catecholaminergic neurons are unique in that they are equipped with a high affinity pump that will sequester the amines back into the axon. The uptake of these byproducts is sodium dependent. To demonstrate the importance of this system cocaine can be administered to the nerve endings and the resultant increase in synaptic amines will be evident as the reuptake of these amines is inhibited. The system of norepinepherine transport has been cloned and is sodium dependent. The structure of this pump is a 617 amino acid structure with 12 hydrophobic amino acid sequences spanning the membrane.

Degradation of the catecholamine neurotransmitters is accomplished by two enzymes, catechol-O-methyltransferase and monoamine oxidase. These are abbreviated using COMT & MAO. Norepinepherine is reacted with MAO to yield dihydroxyphenylglycoaldehyde. If this is then reacted with dehydrogenase, it yields 3'4' dehydroxymandelic acid, or if it is reacted with aldehyde reductase it yields 3'4'dihydroxyphenol-ethyl-glycol. If norepinepherine is reacted with COMT it will yield Normetanepherine. COMT attaches a methyl group to the ring while MAO oxidizes the amine portion of the amine. The metabolites are measured in the urine of patients suspected of adrenal tumor called pheochromocytoma.

MAO is found intracellularly within the mitochondrial membranes of glial cells and neurons in the brain, liver, kidneys, glandular tissue and intestinal tissue. The distribution of the enzyme is suggestive of its role in the metabolism of toxic substances. The evidence of this suggestion comes from the pharmacologic inhibition that occurs in depressive diseases. Tyranamine absorption from the GI tract increases and produces increased release of the sympathetic nervous system that may lead to hypertensive crisis and possible death. The tyranamine is normally oxidized by the enzyme MAO. MAO is a substance commonly found in cheese and wine, which can have potentially fatal consequences. It has a molecular weight of 102,000kd and comes in two subtypes, MAO-A and MAO-B. The newest theory of treating depressive disorders is the inhibition of this enzyme. By inhibiting this enzyme, there are more biogenic amines to be made available to the receptors so that you can counter act the depressive disease. It is important to note that the action of this enzyme is the oxidation of the amines to the respective aldehydes. The product of the degradation of norepinepherine and epinephrine when reacted with MAO is dihydroxyphenylglycoaldehyde. This can be reacted with two enzymes to yield two different products, DOPEG and DOMA, depending on the enzyme acting in the reaction. If this product is reacted with the enzyme Catechol-O-methyl transferase, the end product yields two different 3 methoxy derivatives. These derivatives are 3'methoxy-4'hydroxyphenolethylglycol (MHPG) and vanillymasndelic acid (VMA). It is the urinary analysis of these two byproducts especially VMA that is used in the diagnosis of autonomic system disorders. There is evidence to show that the aldehyde reductase pathway is the most active in the central nervous system. This is due to the increased MHPG or DHPG seen with increased noradrenergic or adrenergic activity. The primary metabolic byproduct if MAO reaction with central dopamine is dihydorxyphenylacetic acid. If this product is then reacted with COMT, it will yield homovanillic acid (HVA). COMT is a cytoplasmic enzyme. The molecular weight of this enzyme is 24,000kd. S-adenosylmethionine plus a divalent cation Mg 2+ are required to activate the enzyme as cofactors. The action of the enzyme is the transfer of a methyl group from SAM to the 3-hydroxy group of the catecholamine. COMT is also able to methylate the catechol containing drugs like isoproterenol. COMT will yield metanepherine, normetanepherine or 3-methoxytyranamine when reacted with epinephrine, norepinepherine, or dopamine.

Dopamine was originally thought to only be a precursor of the norepinepherine and epinephrine transmitters. Recent experimental evidence has shown that dopamine accounts for almost 50% of the catecholamines within the mammalian brain. In the peripheral autonomic ganglia, the dopaminergic nerves are seen as interneurons. Similar very short axons are seen in the retina and the olfactory bulbs. The functions of these are for the modification of sensory inputs. In the retina, it is called lateral inhibition. This is very important in the processing of visual information. Intermediate length interneurons that are dopaminergic in cytology are found in the tuberoinfindibular and hypophysial, incertohypothalamic and medullary periventricular groups. The tuberoinfindibular nerves have a neurohumoral function. They secrete dopamine in to the portal circulation to supply the anterior pituitary. The release of prolactin is directly related to the amount of the dopamine released into the circulation. Dopamine inhibits the secretion of the releasing hormones required for the release of prolactin. Axons that originate from the substantia nigra and the ventral tegmentum are long axons that innervate the basal ganglia, the limbic system, and the frontal cortex. The neostriatial system has cell bodies within the substantia nigra that innervate the caudate and the putamen. It is from these paths that the conclusion is drawn that dopamine has a motor function as released from the neostriatial regions. Parkinson's patients show a decreased release of dopamine from these areas. L-Dopa has the ability to bypass the tyrosine hydroxylase reaction to resolve some of the aforementioned motor problems seen with this disorder.

Serotonin is another of the line of neurotransmitters that parallel the function of norepinepherine within the brain. Serotonin is an indolamine that is synthesized from the essential amino acid tryptophan. There is a specialized transport pump that transports the aromatic and branched chain amino acids across the blood brain barrier. It stands to reason that the concentration of tryptophan will then have implications on the levels of serotonin. The levels of this neurotransmitter can be altered by dietary intake. Tryptophan is hydroxylated by tryptophan hydroxylase found within the serotoninergic nerves. This enzyme, like tyrosine hydroxylase utilized molecular oxygen and tetrahydrobiopterin as a cofactor. The synthesis of serotonin begins with tryptophan that is reacted with tryptophan hydroxylase to yield 5 hydroxytryptophan. This product will then be reacted with the enzyme L-amino acid decarboxylase to produce serotonin. Regulation of this enzyme is somewhat different from the related family of enzymes. Phosphorylation, calcium, phospholipids and partial proteolysis act as regulators for this enzyme. This enzyme is not regulated by end product inhibition as is the case with tyrosine hydroxylase. Dopamine or norepinepherine are feed back inhibited, but the same is not true for serotonin. Evidence of this is seen with the action of MAO on neurotransmitters, catecholamine synthesis will decrease dramatically but the synthesis of serotonin will increase by 300%. The second step in the synthesis of serotonin is the decarboxylation of 5 hydroxytryptophan. This decarboxylation mimics the decarboxylation that produces dopamine from L-Dopa. This however, is not the rate limiting step in the synthesis of serotonin. Serotonin is actively uptaken and stored in granules at the nerve terminals. Theses granules are specific to the transmitter and the pumps that are responsible for the uptake are able to be inhibited by the drug reserpine. If inhibition of the uptake of serotonin occurs, then inhibition of all four biogenic amines is likewise inhibited.

Degradation of serotonin is accomplished by the enzyme MAO. This enzyme regulates the uptake of the transmitter into the nerve terminals and degradation. There is a difference in the ring structure of the indolamines when compared to the catecholamines. It is this difference that creates a differing pathway or each. Serotonin degradation begins with serotonin being reacted with MAO; the product is 5 hydroxyindole acetaldehyde. This product can be reacted on by two enzymes aldehyde reductase to yield 5 hydrotryptophol. The second part of this reaction is the reaction of the dehydrogenase on the same intermediate that will yield 5 hydroxyindole acetate acid (5HIAA). The oxidation of the indolamine to 5 hydroxyindole acetic acid via the intermediate indoleeacealdehyde occurs using NAD as a cofactor.

Histamine is another transmitter found in the brain of mammals and in Mast cells. Histamine is also an imidazole containing substance. The enzyme responsible for the synthesis of histamine is Histidine decarboxylase. This enzyme is very similar to amino acid decarboxylase that produces catecholamines and serotonin. Histamine is produced by the decarboxylation of the essential amino acid histamine. The enzyme histadine decarboxylase has been isolated in the fetal liver and is similar in its actions in the central nervous system. Like most decarboxylases, this enzyme requires Vitamin B6 as a cofactor. This enzyme rarely saturates and can be affected by the dietary intake of the essential amino acid. It is possible to increase the amount of histamine in the brain via histadine loading.

Like tryptophan hydroxylase, the affinity (Km) for histadine decarboxylase is higher than the amount of substrate available for possible decarboxylation. The major catabolic pathway for the elimination of histamine is via the N-methylation to methylhistamine. The enzyme responsible for this reaction is histamine methyltransferase. The cofactor required for this reaction is S-adenosylmethionine, which donates a methyl group. The enzyme MAO will react on the product methylhistamine to be further catabolized. Research has uncovered nerve pathways that originate in the posterior basal hypothalamus and premamillary areas using the introduction of histamine decarboxylase antibodies. This is the basis of the experimental models set forth in newer studies of the midbrain.

Gamma-Aminobutyric acid is another neurotransmitter found within the brain. The function of this transmitter is in the transmission of impulses for the internal circuits of very specific areas of the brain, spinal cord, and the retina. The reaction that takes glutamate to being GABA is a decarboxylation reaction. The enzyme responsible for this decarboxylation is glutamic acid decarboxylase (GAD). This reaction involves the removal of the alpha carboxyl to yield gamma carboxyl. The cofactor required is vitamin B6 (pyridol phosphate). The manner of rate limiting is also unique in that it is accomplished by the saturation of GAD with B6. Additional control is found with the steric hindrance associated with ATP. This would explain the increase in this neurotransmitter by 30-45% postmortem when the ATP levels drop. GAD is very selective in the areas it is found within the brain. This enzyme is not seen in glia or in other types of neurons. GABA is synthesized from alpha-oxogluterate through glutamate. GABA is degraded via two enzymes that allow the end product to be returned to the Krebs's cycle as succinic acid. The GABA shunt is specific to the brain and constitutes a viable source of energy for the brain. This energy source contributes 10-40% of the brain's metabolism. Also, glial cells contain a high affinity pump for GABA. These pumps function to seek out the GABA and utilize it for energy. The GABA that is degraded in the GABAergic nerves allows for the regeneration of glutamate. The enzyme GAD is highly concentrated in areas that are high in GABA, but the actual GABA degrading enzymes, GABA transaminase, succinic semialdehyde dehydrogenase are found throughout the brain. The reactions that are involved in the synthesis and degradation of GBA include the synthesis of GABA by the enzyme GABA transaminase to yield succinic semialdehyde which is then put back into the Krebs's cycle will also elicit the regeneration of glutamate from oxogluterate. The succinic semialdehyde is put back into the Krebs's cycle by the action of succinic semialdehydedehydrogenase or it can be degraded to alpha-hydroxybutyrate. The driving mechanism behind this reaction is glucose. The catabolism of GABA is terminated by the uptake and recycling of the transmitter into glutamate and ATP. This uptake requires an active transport and the structure of this transport protein is a large protein with 12 membrane spanning domains. These domains are made up of hydrophobic amino acids that can be inserted into the lipid bilayer. The transport is sodium dependent and takes 2 sodium molecules to drive 1 GABA and 1 chloride molecule. GABA is metabolized by several enzymes throughout the brain. The cofactor for this degradation is Vitamin B6 and it associates with the enzyme GABA transaminase. The enzyme will compete with GAD at certain times for the receptor site. This is the reason that we see seizure activity with B6 Deficiency. The transamination of GABA to succinic semialdehyde by GABA transaminase produces the glutamate that will be decarboxylated to become GABA that will act as an inhibitor in conjunction with Chloride. This occurs via the hypopolarization of the nerve in response to the uptake of GABA and Chloride.

CHAPTER 9

SYNAPTIC TRANSMISSION

The cells of the nervous system are like cells of almost every other system in that they must communicate with each other and the surrounding environment in order to function. In the human nervous system, the basic pretext of the system is the ability to accept input information from the internal and external environment and transfer that information into communicable impulses. Within the system, the electrical signaling is transferred at specific points termed the synapses. The structure and function of the synapse is dynamic. Neuroscientists' understanding of the synapse has grown tremendously in the past 20 years. In the human nervous system, the communication that is required for effective functioning is of extreme speed. In order for this aspect of the nervous system to work there must be some functional or structural methodology that will allow for this extremely rapid communication. Within the body there are many examples of the body's ability to communicate cell to cell. Identification of this cell to cell communication network has been well studied and well documented. The connexon junction and the cardiac myocytes are just two examples of such cell to cell communication situations. The signaling that is seen in the body is either of a chemical or electrical nature. There are aspects of each type of signaling that are structural and others that are functional that will distinguish one from another.

Properties of Signaling Mechanisms.

CHEMICAL SIGNALING	ELECTRICAL SIGNALING
Must use chemical transmitter	Fewer numbers
Very plastic	Generally seen in short acting signal
Great ability to act as amplifiers	Generally not inhibitor signals
Generally see in higher functions of the nervous system	Very extreme speed of transmission

In the electrical signaling system, there are ion channels that will allow the flow of the current and thus allow the signaling connection between the pre and the post synaptic cell. In the electrical signaling system, this signal is able to be transmitted in both a unidirectional or bidirectional manner. In the electrical signaling system, the ion channel of the presynaptic cell must be able to complete two specific tasks. They must be able to create the depolarization of the presynaptic membrane and generate an action potential and they must also be able to pass that current to the post synaptic cell.

Characteristics of Chemical synapses versus Electrical synapses

Distance Btn pre—& post	30-50 nm	3.5nm
Is there cytoplasmic continuity between the pre-& post	No	Yes
Method of transmission	Active zones & post receptors	Gap Junctions
How transmission occurs	Chemical	Ionic
Directional regulation	Unidirectional	Bidirectional

The expressed benefit of the electrical signal model is the extremely rapid transmission of the signal. This speed of transmission is due to the direct flow of the ions from the presynaptic cell to the postsynaptic cell. In many parts of the nervous system, the electrical signaling is not just a cell to cell communication, but rather these signaling cells have the ability to communicate with groups of neurons. This ability for the communication of groups of neurons is the basis of the syncitial activity of tissues like the heart. This property discloses something about the actual physical property of the membranes involved. Ohm's law ($\Delta V = \Delta I \text{ x } R$) states that the lower the resistance of the neuron (R), the smaller the depolarization (V) that will be required by the incoming stimulus (ΔI) to push the threshold over the required value to generate the action potential and thus create the synchronous excitation of the cell group.

The numbers of electrical signaling type of communication that is seen in those aspects of higher function such as learning and memory has been demonstrated experimentally and confirmed by a number of other authors. The prevailing theory for the specific function of this signal type in these higher functions is the actual structure of the signaling mechanism itself. It is believed that the size of the gap junction is responsible for this property of the neuronal signalling. The size of this channel is approximately 1.5 nm. The size of the gap junction will allow the transport of molecules with molar weights of slightly greater than 1000 Kda.

The gap junction that is responsible for this transmission of molecules is a non rectifying synapse. The gap junction is also responsible for the directional flow of the ions that are responsible for the generation of the action potential. As mentioned previously, the capacity exists for the impulse to be transmitted bidirectionally, however the histologic structure maintains unidirectional transmission in most instances. The structure of the gap junction is such that there are two distinct parts of the channel. The structure is composed of a pair of hemi channels with one pair being presynaptic and the remaining pair being post synaptic. The descriptive names of pre and post synaptic indicate that the two membranes are separated by a space. This space is called a gap and therefore the name gap junction exists. The two separate membranes are connected by the chemical interaction. The hemi cylinders are themselves called a connexon. The connexon is further subdivided into six identical protein subunits. These subunits are called connexins. The connexon is identified as being hexagonally arranged in lengths of approximately 7.5 nm.

The connexin has a specific function as well for it is the part of the hemi channel that will recognize the opposing connexon. It is the two opposing connexin that will join functionally and form a connexon. The other function that is bestowed upon the connexin is that of auto-recognition. It has the responsibility of recognizing the other five protein subunits that are destined to lie adjacent to the protein and form the connexon entity. If this recognition does not occur, then there is no formation of a connexon and no channel formation and therefore no ion transfer and no action potential propagation.

The function of the gap junction is unique in that it opens by a conformational change in the structure of the channel itself. On opening the channel the proteins that constitute the connexon will rotate slightly to increase the opening of the interior of the channel and allow the ions to flow through. The interior or the cytoplasmic regions of the channel are variable in the amino acid sequencing that dictates the structure and the function of the channel. This is in stark contrast to the transmembrane sequences that are known to be of only four hydrophobic domains with each chain being highly conserved from cell to cell. The cytoplasmic variations are the rationale behind the theory of the variability of different tissues sensitivity to a variety of modulatory substances.

The other type of signaling that is seen in the humans nervous system is the chemical synapse. In this type of synapse, the pre and the post synaptic membranes are also separated by a gap between the cell membranes. This synaptic cleft is significantly wider than those mentioned in the electrical signaling system. In the chemical signaling system, the synaptic cleft is approximately 20-40 nm wide. In the pre-synaptic membrane there are specialized regions and those regions have very specialized functions. The action potential that is propagated along the presynaptic axon to the terminal will initiate a cascade of events that will induce a release of neurotransmitter that will pass across the synaptic cleft to create a post synaptic effect. These steps are the rationale for the slowed speed of transmission that is inherent in the chemical signaling versus the electrical signaling.

In the presynaptic terminal there are as mentioned previously, specialized areas that will perform specialized functions. One such area is the active zone. The active zone is found presynaptically at the terminal portion of the presynaptic neuron. The function of the active zone is the release of the packaged neurotransmitter chemicals into the space between the pre and the post synaptic membranes, AKA, the synaptic cleft. There are some neurons that do not have these active zones. The substance that is released is called a neurotransmitter. This substance can have variable effects and methods of action. Typical models of the relationship between the neurotransmitter and the synapse will have the neurotransmitter exerting its effect on the directly opposing cell or directly adjacent cells. In other models the neurotransmitter can be a modulator. In certain instances, the neurotransmitter can be released into the blood and exert its effect at a distant point. The idea of a neurohormones is defined by this property of neurotransmitters.

In the chemical signaling system, the action of the neurotransmitter is dependent upon the post synaptic receptor and the properties of that membrane. It is the postsynaptic receptor that will dictate the effect of the cholinergic neurotransmitter is an excitatory or inhibitory effect. This receptor on the post synaptic aspect is also responsible for the inclusion of possible second messenger systems for signal amplification or if the neurotransmitter is to exert its effect directly. So if the post synaptic receptor is the deciding factor, then all post synaptic receptors must be alike. From a morphologic standpoint, there are two basic biochemical principles that are common with all post synaptic receptors. One is that they are all membrane spanning proteins. The extracellular side of the membrane protein is responsible for the actual recognition and binding of the neurotransmitter from the presynaptic cell. Second, is that they will exert an effect on the post synaptic cell. This effect is possible to be exerted directly or indirectly, or even by the activation of a second messenger system. Classification of the signaling systems are that these receptors are either direct or indirect in the method they gate the ions as they are transported across the cell channel.

There are many receptors that have been investigated in the human nervous system, but those with the direct activation and therefore direct flow of ions, like those that mediate the acetylcholine neurotransmitter are generally single polypeptide chains. These directly activated channels are of such a nature that they undergo a conformational change in the protein subunits with the binding of the neurotransmitter. This conformational change allows for the passage of the macromolecules as the channel is in the open position. Neurotransmitters that act via channels like this are the ones for glycine, GABA and glutamate.

Receptors that are able to act via an indirect method are those for norepinepherine and serotonin. In this type of receptor, the binding is to a receptor that will initiate a cascade of events that will, through the use of a G-coupled protein, act on a second messenger to exert the effects of the neurotransmitter. The protein associated with this process is guanosine Triphosphate that will bind to the receptor and to the effector enzyme. This binding to the effector enzyme will initiate a signal within the cell using the "second messenger system." The second messenger system will utilize cyclic adenosine monophosphate (cAMP) or diacylglycerol (DAG). This second messenger system works via one of two possible pathways. In the first path, the action is direct on the channel. The more commonly seen alternative is the activation of a second family of enzymes called protein kinases that will either activate by phospohrylation of the channel directly of phosphorylation of a modulating protein to exert its effect on the ion channel.

Because of the properties mentioned above, the chemical signaling is divided into two distinct processes. The first process is that of the release of the chemical transmitter and therefore the process is that of the transmission of the action potential. The second process is the reception of the chemical signal from the pre synaptic membrane. The process is found within the post synaptic membrane and it is the process of receiving the chemical signal. The chemical signaling process is a complex one and has many steps that are involved in the entirety of the process. It has been said the presynaptic aspect of the process is analogous to the functioning of an endocrine gland.

The theory that the system is static and uncompromising no longer holds true. Vast experimental evidence has demonstrated the ability of the system, especially the synaptic communication to be dynamic or in the neuroscientists' language, having the property of neural plasticity. There is an ability of the synapse to be "plastic", or have the ability to modify itself. These plastic modifications are not limited to shape alone. Plasticity also refers to the ability of the system to increase in numbers, connectivity, shape and size.

In order to better understand the nature of the signaling that is accomplished via the nervous system, a better understanding of the actual structures that are involved in synaptic transmission will be undertaken at this point. Synapses are not a single component, but rather a multiple component structure. The complexity of the synaptic structures has been the premise for many researchers through history, and because of those efforts our understanding of these important cytoarcheticetural structures has expanded tremendously. The synapse is composed of presynaptic structures and post synaptic structures. The architecture of the synapse is unique in the structure of the presynaptic component containing small clear synaptic vessicles, approximately 40nm in diameter. These synaptic vessicles contain the neurotransmitter specific for that synapse. Additional distinguishing factors are the increased numbers of mitochondria located within the presynaptic aspect of the synapse. There are also very dense cored vessicles that are found to contain neuropeptides that are transported from the soma or other vessicles that are found to contain the catecholamines synthesized within the synaptic terminal. The postsynaptic aspect of the synapse is in direct physical opposition of the presynaptic portion.

The complexity of the nervous system is evident in the manner the presynaptic aspect of the synapse functions. The speed with which the terminal must be ready to propagate the action potential and convert this into chemical release is measured in milliseconds. Therefore there must be a mechanism for the rapid conversion of this electrical impulse into the chemical neurotransmitter released into the synaptic cleft. The property of axonal transport is well understood and demonstrated. In antegrade transport, the terminal has the ability to replenish the constituents of the neurotransmitter formed at the presynaptic terminal, the molecular proteins required for the structural integrity of the terminal and other substances that the terminal may require. In the case of the fast antegrade transport, the speed of this transport is only 200-400 mm/day. This is not consistent with the requirements of supporting the possible 1-100m/sec speed of the action potential. Therefore there must be a different mechanism of provision of the material of the presynaptic membrane to provide the components of the neurotransmitter required for the propagation of the action potential along through the synaptic cleft to the post synaptic membrane. In order for this speed to be accommodated there must be a storage mechanism of the neurotransmitter components or the neurotransmitters themselves within the presynaptic membrane. Experimental evidence suggests that this is in fact the situation, at least in part.

The presynaptic terminal is somewhat sufficient in its ability to sustain itself. The terminal does not have the ability to store all the enzymes that are required for the synthesis of many of the membrane proteins that are need to be incorporated into the synaptic vessicles. These proteins that are lacking must then be transported from the soma. The neurotransmitters, mainly acetylcholine, are released from the vessicles described but there is also evidence of non-vessicle release of neurotransmitter. This discussion will focus on the vessicle released neurotransmitters. The amount of neurotransmitter released from the presynaptic terminal is a relatively constant amount. The release of this acetylcholine in amounts defined as quanta, a relatively consistent amount of 10,000 vessicles is released concurrently. A Quanta, is defined as the equivalent number of neurotransmitter molecules found within each vessicle. The synaptic vessicle is located at very precise locations within the presynaptic membrane. This particular point is called the active zone. It is such a precise location due to the attachment of the vessicle to the membrane by actin filaments. The actin is attached to the synaptic vessicle by a second protein called synapsin. It is therefore the synapsin that is the protein actually contacting the vessicle. Additional to the protein attachment there is an increased number of voltage sensitive calcium channels localized around the active zone. Since the depolarization of the axon terminal produces increased localization of calcium influx, this increased calcium will bind to the plasma membrane to stimulate the exocytosis of the neurotransmitter. For the vessicle to be released into the synaptic cleft there must be a disengagement of the synapsin from the vessicle. For the release of the vessicle there is a phosphorylation of the synapsin that will provide the energy required for this disengagement. This does not produce immediate release into the synaptic cleft but rather it allows the vessicle to move "down line" towards the membrane. Once there is contact with the membrane, there appears to be a conformational change that creates a fusion of the vesicle to the membrane. This fusion allows for the release of the neurotransmitter within the vessicle.

It is thought there are two differing pathways for the two types of vessicles, one for the clear vessicles and a second pathway for the neurosecretory vesicles. The neurosecretory vesicles are not concentrated near the active zones as are the clear vesicles. The necessity for the neurosecretory vesicles to be located near the active zone is negated due to the reduced concentration of calcium that is required for the activation of the release mechanism. There is an additional component in the release mechanism as well. In the neurosecretory vesicle, there is a higher frequency of stimulation required to activate the release. Experimental data has demonstrated that the release of the clear vesicle to be phasic in nature. This is in contrast to the constant release demonstrated by the neurosecretory vesicle.

Once released from the presynaptic membrane, the neurotransmitter is passed into the synaptic cleft in its journey to the postsynaptic membrane. Once released into the synaptic cleft, the neurotransmitter is acted upon by a variety of enzymes that will modify the chemical composition of the transmitter. The process of this journey across the cleft is not a simple one either. There are two types of synaptic transmission seen in the human nervous system. In the diffusion of the neurotransmitter across the cleft the time of diffusion can be very rapid as is the case for the neuromuscular junction. In this situation the time of diffusion is only 50 μ sec from presynaptic membrane to postsynaptic membrane. The total delay time from presynaptic release to postsynaptic receptor is variable and dependent upon the transduction mechanism of the postsynaptic membrane.

In the fast chemical neurotransmission, there is a total delay that is measured in milliseconds as opposed to the total delay seen in the slow chemical neurotransmission which demonstrates a time of hundreds of milliseconds. In the situation of the fast chemical transmission the structure of the postsynaptic receptor is an ion channel. Since this is an ion channel, only smaller sized neurotransmitters, Na+, K+, Ca++, Cl- are able to be bound and accepted. The most common name for this type of transmission is the “ligand gated / receptor gated ion channel”. Since these molecules are ions they create alteration in the transmembrane electrical potential, an action potential, IPSP or EPSP.

In slow chemical transmission, the mechanism of the transmission involves G proteins. This is a very slow process as the G protein must then couple to the receptor and initiate the cascade. In this situation, the cell that is acted upon is a neuropeptide. Once it is bound by the G protein, the activation of the neuropeptide will then acts upon and activate an enzyme to elicit its intracellular effect. The intracellular effect is to activate cyclic AMP, a second messenger. Once the cAMP is activated there is a wide variety of secondary effects that will be induced in the effector.

Synaptic transmission is not a random or haphazard process. The propagation of the impulses involved in the action potential involves eight very specific functions. These functions include:

- The synthesis of the secretory vesicles within the soma and then transported to the synaptic terminal.
- The vesicle must be filled with the neurotransmitter. In the case where the neurotransmitter is a neuropeptide, the filling of the vesicle is completed as the vesicle is formed.
- The presynaptic terminal must receive the depolarization
- The synaptic vesicle must be attached through the protein synapsin to the presynaptic membrane.
- There must be the exocytosis of the neurotransmitter into the synaptic cleft.
- There must be the diffusion of the neurotransmitter across the synaptic cleft and it must then bind to the postsynaptic receptor.

- There must be a postsynaptic response elicited from the binding of the neurotransmitter to the postsynaptic membrane receptor.
- There must be an active reuptake by the presynaptic membrane of the vesicle and any additional neurotransmitter.
- There must be some form of degradation of the additional neurotransmitter within the synaptic cleft.

In many synapses, the amount of the neurotransmitter that is released is proportional to the amplitude of the action potential.

What is a synaptic vesicle? Synaptic vesicles are similar to the cellular membrane we are all familiar with. Synaptic vesicles are made from a lipid bilayer with the same type of transmembrane proteins that are seen in conventional cell membranes. The architecture of the membrane is composed of the same channels as are seen in the conventional cell membrane, they form calcium channels and like structural support. There are also likenesses between the dense core vesicles and the synaptic vesicles. The common protein composition is how they both contain synaptotagmin and SV2 proteins. Within the synaptic vesicle, there are increased amounts of the proteins synaptophysin and synaptobrevin.

Within the synaptic vesicle there are several types of transporters for the neurotransmitter. These are the protein coupled transporters. These transport proteins are specific for the neurotransmitters. One protein coupled transporter is available for the biogenic amines, another is for acetylcholine, and another is for glutamate and another for Glycine / GABA. It is the specificity of these protein coupled transporters that allows the rapid influx of the neurotransmitters required for action potential propagation.

On the postsynaptic side of the structure called the synaptic cleft, the membrane will have very specific target receptor molecules. These target molecules are transmembrane proteins, specifically glycoproteins that will allow for the binding of the neurotransmitter. The receptors are named according to the neurotransmitter that they bind. If the receptor binds acetylcholine, they are called cholinergic receptors. These receptors can be further subdivided into nicotinic and muscarinic receptor subtypes. The nicotinic receptor is generally an excitatory receptor while the muscarinic are generally inhibitory in function. Muscarinic receptors can be further subclassification with M1 thru M5 muscarinic subtypes. If the receptor binds catecholamines like epinephrine or norepinepherine, they are then called adrenergic. The adrenergic receptors are also subdivided into the α and β receptors. These are further subdivided into the α1, α2, α3 or the β1, β2, β3 receptors.

The membrane coupled receptors are of two classifications, either the ligand gated ion channels or the G protein coupled receptors. The ligand gated ion channel is a transmembranous glycoprotein that spans the postsynaptic cell membrane. There are two subclassification of the ligand gated ion channel, those that are nicotinic cholinergic, the serotonin, those that are the GABA and Glycine receptor family and the second family that is for the excitatory glutamate family. The G protein family is by far the larger of the two families. 75% of the chemical messengers will exert their effect via the G protein coupled receptors. In the G protein coupled receptor, the structural make up of this receptor is the exterior aspect of the receptor is exposed to the outer membrane and the internal aspect of the complex is composed of the guanosine triphosphate binding protein and the effector protein. The actual guanosine triphosphate binding protein is composed of the α, β, and γ subunits. Because of the complexity of the unit as a whole the action of this second messenger system is very slow to initiate the effector response.

Deeper investigation of the chemical synapses will demonstrate that they are the predominant signaling method of the human brain. As discussed above the two types of this chemical signaling are the directly gated ion channel and the indirectly gated or the second messenger model of signal transmission. The best understood of the directly gated ion channels are the motor end plates of skeletal muscle. In this type of ion channel or synaptic arrangement, the neurotransmitter involved is acetylcholine or ACh. In this model, a single muscle fiber is innervated by one motor neuron. In this model, the neurotransmitter that will be released will follow the description previously mentioned, using ACh as the transmitter and the receptor will be one specific for acetylcholine, the ACh nicotinic receptor. The activation of the receptor is designed to excite the specialized region of the post synaptic membrane called the motor end plate. The end plate is generally a slight depression in the post synaptic membrane of the muscle fiber. The structure of this area is very unique as well. The insulation covering of the nerve is called myelin and as the end plate is found along it borders, the myelin sheath disappears. The axon will continue in progression from larger diameter axon into very small projections that are fiber like, these individual fiber like projections are termed the synaptic boutons. It is within the tips of the synaptic boutons that the actual neurotransmitter is released from. The synaptic boutons are seen to lie above the post synaptic membrane and the junctional folds present in the post synaptic membrane. These junctional folds are designed to increase the surface are of the post synaptic membrane and therefore increase the number of receptors available for binding of the neurotransmitter that has been released from the pre synaptic terminal boutons.

The synaptic boutons are the site of the release of the synaptic vesicles that contain the neurotransmitter ACh. Also included in the synaptic bouton will be the active zone and the voltage gated calcium channel. It is at the active zone where the calcium is uptaken to assist in the fusion that is required to have the synaptic vesicle fuse with the membrane for its impending release. It is important to understand that each active zone is opposed by a postsynaptic junctional fold. This is important as the concentration of the receptors located at this region of the junctional fold have been experimentally demonstrated to be around 10,000 receptors per μm. The region is in contrast to the increased concentration to the voltage gated sodium channels that are demonstrated to lie within the bottom of the folds. It is the voltage gated sodium channels that are responsible for the conversion of the endplate potential into the propagated action potential. The conversion is due to the opening of the ACh containing synaptic vesicles.

Second messenger systems are so named because once the neurotransmitter binds and elicits its effects; the effects are carried out through a series of additional molecules. In this type of molecular signaling the receptor is much more important as it will play a much more complex role. Upon the binding of the specific neurotransmitter, the receptor will elicit a change on the biochemistry of the cell. The complexity of this process is evidenced by the mechanisms they exert their actions upon the cell. One class of receptor, the action is exerted directly on the cell, and on the other class of receptor, the action is exerted via a coupled receptor. These receptors are known to utilize an indirect method of activity. In majority of the synaptic activity, there is a gated ion that will most often utilize G proteins (GTP). Owing to the use of this second messenger method of activity, the effects of this transmission type are slower in eliciting final activity but amplified in the amount of molecular transmitter required for a more global activation. Structurally, these second messenger channels are different as well. These receptors are seen to consist of a single polypeptide chain rather than the multiple chains that have been identified in directly activating channels. The activation of the channel is important for differing cellular functions and durations. As was mentioned previously, the second messenger synaptic transmission has prolonged effectiveness but this comes about with the sacrifice of speed of activation. Experimental evidence has demonstrated a common genetic familial connection between all of the second messenger receptor proteins. We also know that the use of cAMP (cyclic adenosine monophosphate), inositol polyphosphate or diacylglycerol (DAG) are commonly used as second messenger coupling molecules. It has also been demonstrated that in certain instance, metabolites are capable of acting as the second messenger. Examples of this are arachnadonic acid. The second messenger pathways require the activation of a kinase enzyme to create the opening or the closing of the channel or activating the calcium ions within the cell. These pathways are not mutually exclusive in nature, rather in many instance these pathways are mutually beneficial. The definition of this component is often referred to as "cross-talk" between the pathways. This functional characteristic is due to the ability of many proteins to be modified at multiple sites within the same protein. The best understood of these multi-modified receptors are the synapsin I and the ***B*** adrenergic receptor proteins. Therefore, the process is more complex and greater possibility for perturbation. This can be a positive aspect from a pharmacologic point of view.

CHAPTER 10

THE MENINGES

The meninges are the membranous coverings of the central nervous system. They are found deep to the hard bony covering called the skull and the bony cover of the spinal cord, the vertebral column. The meninges serve two specific functions. The first function of the meninges is to add to the protection of the brain and the spinal cord. The second function of the meninges is to provide a supportive framework for the neural tissue by providing a framework for the venous structures, arteries and sinuses. There is a space contained within the meninges that is a fluid filled space. This space is called the subarachnoid space. The meninges are actually a collection of tissue, the dura mater, the pia mater and the arachnoid. The word mater is derived from the Greek word for mother.

The meninges will develop form the neural crest cells and the mesenchyme or the mesoderm. These cells will migrate from the neural crest to eventually surround the developing nervous system within 25-30 days. The immature neural crest cells and the mesoderm are collectively called the primitive meninges or the meninx primitive. During this point of the developing nervous system, there is no subarachnoid space. The primitive meninges will begin to differentiate at around day 34-48 of gestation. After this differentiation is complete there are specific layers that ectomeninix will continue to differentiate and will become apparent. The compact outer layer also known as the ectomeninix and the endomeninix, a reticulated layer will develop from the differentiation of the developing mesoderm. The developing meninges will continue to mature and differentiate such that at gestational day 45-60 the beginnings of the venous structures will become identifiable. The endomeninix will become more reticulated and the cisterns will become identifiable. The same is true for the subarachnoid space. It begins to become discernable in its structure. As the differentiation continues, the ectomeninix will eventually become the dura mater. The endomeninix will differentiate significantly more than the ectomeninix in that it will become the pia mater and the arachnoid. The time frame of this differentiation is very important since the majority of the development of the meninges will be completed by the completion of the first trimester.

This development is slightly different within the cranial vault. The skeletal layer of the ectomeninix will actually form the skull. This arrangement of fibers is how the adult remnants will have fibers that attach the dura to the inside plate of the periosteum. In the spinal canal, the differentiation is the same but there develops a potential space that will become the epidural space. From a histologic standpoint, the predominant cell type of the meninges is a fibroblast. In tissue section with H&E staining, the majority of cell type identification is large elongated fibroblasts. It is commonly referred to as the pachymeninix. Interspersed within the elongated fibroblasts are many collagen fibrils.

The overall structure of the meninges is that it consists of three layers, the dura mater, the arachnoid mater, and the pia mater. As mentioned above, the outer layer the dura mater is attached to the bone of the skull and the spinal cord via remnant structures called the denticulate ligaments. Moving deeper, the next layer is the arachnoid layer. It is called the arachnoid because it resembles a spider's web. The arachnoid layer is complex in structure yet it can yield a strong yet flexible attachment for the neural tissue to the bone. The arachnoid is separated from the inner pia mater by the subarachnoid space. The subarachnoid space contains cerebrospinal fluid, and vascular structures. Traversing the subarachnoid space are fibroblasts that are identified histologically. It is important to identify these cells because they are the lionshare of the actual subarachnoid trabeculae. Closer inspection of the subarachnoid space yields neither direct nerve endings nor any direct vascular supply. So the arachnoid is avascular and void of innervation. These characteristics present unusual problems when there is trauma or other pathologic conditions that are presented as an insult to the bone- dura- neural structures.

As one continues to penetrate deeper in the meningeal layers the structure identified is the pia mater. It is the most delicate and yet the most intimate layer of the meningeal coverings. It is such an intimate fit that the pia follows every invagination and elevation of the brain and spinal cord. The pia mater will give rise to the rigid structural separations of the brain. This is the engineering feat of the pia mater. Its outer aspects provide a mobile yet very strong attachment and the inner aspects create rigid points of separation. These separations are structures like the falx cerebri. The actual structural attachment of the spinal cord is itself composed of remnant pia mater. The Filum terminale is histologically identical to the consistency of the pial layer. It serves as anatomic reference as well as functional attachment of the spinal cord during embryologic development and continuing through adult life. In many texts the pia and the arachnoid are together called the leptomeninges. The dura is a membrane that is actually subdivided into 3 layers. There is an outer periosteal layer an inner meningeal layer and a border cell layer. The differentiation of the outer periosteal layer is in the histology of the fibroblasts. In the periosteal layer, the fibroblasts are less elongated and packed with a greater density. This is especially true along the suture lines of the skull and at the base of the skull. There is a greater concentration of collagen seen in this layer of dura as well when compared to the other dural layers. The dural cell border layer is the innermost of the dural layers and it is composed of flattened fibroblasts. This layer stains for a clear proteoglycan substance but does not stain for collagen or elastin fibers. This is the weakest structural layer of the dura. It is however, contiguous with the meningeal layer and the arachnoid.

The dura folds are made of the periosteal dura. The periosteal dura will differentiate from their normal origin to become the more rigid cells that will invaginate into the neural tissue. These cells will form the falx cerebri and other infoldings. The falx cerebri is the largest of these infoldings. Anatomically, it will attach to the crista galli rostrally and it divides the brain into a right and left hemisphere. Posteriorly and caudally, it will attach to the tentorium cerebelli. At points where these divisions of the dura are found, there are venous structures that occupy these voids. Anatomically, there is the superior sagittal sinus that is found at the junction of the falx cerebri and the skull. There is another venous structure that is found at the point where the falx cerebri attaches to the tentorium cerebelli called the straight sinus. Another venous structure associated with these voids is the inferior sagittal sinus that is seen where the innermost edge of the falx cerebri divides the hemispheres. There is a list of the venous structures that are formed from within the dural infoldings.

Principle Cisterns of the brain

CISTERN	ARTERY	VEIN	CRANIAL NN	STRUCTURE
Ambient	Portions of the posterior cerebral, quadrigeminal & superior cerebellar	Basal vein of Rosenthal	Trochlear	Lateral aspect of the crus cerebri
Cerebellopontine Inferior aka Lateral cereberomedullary	Vertebral & proximal branches of the PICA	Retrooilvary & Lateral medullary	Glossopharyngeal Vagus, Spinal Accessory & hypoglossal	Pyramid, inferior olivary eminence, choroids plexus
Cerebellopontine (superior)	Distal branches of the anterior inferior cerebellar, labyrinthine & basilar	Pontomesencephalic & Petrosal	Trigeminal, Facial & vestibulocochlear	
Chiasmatic	Opthalmic & small branches to the chiasm & hypophysis		Optic NN & optic chiasm	

Cisterna magnum Aka dorsal cerebellomedullary	Distal branches of the PICA & posterior spinal, branches to the choroids plexus of the 4th ventricle	Tonsillar & dorsal medullary		Roots of C1 & C2
Interpenduncular	Rostral end of the basilar AA & portions of the posterior cerebral, choroidal & thalamogeniculate	Portions of the basal VV of Rosenthal	Occulomotor root	Mamillary body & lateral edge of the crus cerebri
Prepontine	Basilar AA & its branches	Pontine VV	Abducens	
Quadrigeminal	Portions of the cerebral, quadrigeminal, choridal AA	Great VV of Galen	Trochlear root	Pineal, superior & inferior Colliculi

The tentorium cerebelli is anatomically the second largest of the dural folds. Upon dissection, it will attach rostrally to the clinoid process. It has a unique tent shape and functions to divide the cranial cavity into the infratentorial and supratentorial compartments. Tissue distribution includes the cerebellum located in the infratentorial region and the occipital lobe lying within the supratentorial region. This division of the cranium into these compartments is important because from a pathologic perspective, one can compartmentalize tumors or infections within the tissue. If a tumor is present, radiologically, identification is made by inspection if the mass displaces the tissue across midline or if it forces the tissue below the tentorium. This is crucial because the structure of the dural folds is rigid enough that space occupying lesions will create necrosis via vascular compromise. If the push of the tissue is severe enough and prolonged enough, death is possible from herniation of the tissue through the foramen magnum. Along the midline of the infratentorial tissue is the falx cerebelli. This dural fold is located within the occipital bone. Along the interior wall of the occipital bone is the occipital sinus and this sinus will empty into the confluence of sinuses.

The smallest of the dural folds is the diapharagma sella. This fold forms the roof of the hypophyseal fossa. It functions to protect the pituitary stalk by encasing the stalk. Inspection of diapharagma sells will relveal the intimate relationship to the sella turcica. The sella turcica will yield a structure that is very unforgiving and obtrusive and yet it affords the maximum protection to the very important pituitary gland and accompanying vascularity. Along the borders of this fold lie the anterior and posterior intercavernous sinuses.

At the margin of the foramen magnum, the periosteal dura ends and the meningeal dura continue. The meningeal dura is seen to follow the entire length of the spinal canal. At the distal termination of the meningeal dura, is the coccygeal ligament. This ligament is a remnant of the dura. It is also called the filum terminale externum. This is the anchor of the spinal tissue to the bony structure.

The arachnoid layer of the dural is deep to the outer dural layer. There are many anatomists that have divided this layer into two sections, the arachnoid barrier cell layer and the arachnoid trabeculae. The arachnoid barrier cell layer is directly apposed to the dural border, while the arachnoid trabeculae traverses the subarachnoid space. The subarachnoid space is located between the arachnoid barrier cell layer and the pial layer. Within this space there are many vessels and more importantly the Cerebrospinal fluid. The arachnoid barrier cell layer is made of predominantly fibroblasts no collagen fibrils to speak of. The arachnoid barrier cell layer is very tenuously attached to the dural border cell layer by occasional cell junctions. In stark contrast, the arachnoid barrier cells have closely apposed sell membranes that are joined by numerous tight junctions. This is the basis for the term barrier cell layer; these tightly joined cells form a barrier that limits the flow of particles and bacteria as well as larger macromolecules.

The arachnoid trabeculae layer and the subarachnoid space are seen to consist of mostly elongated, flattened and irregularly shaped fibroblasts. These fibroblasts are arranged in such a manner as to span the entire width of the subarachnoid space. The most unique aspect of this cellular arrangement is in the strength that is derived from the cytoarchitecture itself. The cellular arrangement is the underlying mechanism of the strength behind this layer of dura. The subarachnoid space is found deep to the barrier cell layer yet superficial to the pia layer. It contains the cerebrospinal fluid, trabeculae cells, collagen, and venous structures. The brain itself is suspended within the cranial vault by the fibers within the subarachnoid space. Anatomists have dispelled the theory that the brain was floating unattached within the CSF. It has been demonstrated that the brain has approximately 97% of its weight by mass suspended within the fluid and that the structure in its whole is anchored slightly by the fibers of the subarachnoid layer. These fibers are what tear with acceleration and deceleration injuries. It is now understood that in diffuse axonal injury, there is some resultant shear that occurs and therefore will produce some tearing of the attachment fibers.

The arachnoid villi have the distinction of extending through the tight cuffs into the sinuses. These villi are found in the meningeal dura along the midline or in cul-du-sacs (lateral or venous lacunae) of the sinuses. If these arachnoid villi are enlarged or calcified that are then called pacchioian bodies. There is uniqueness in the structure of the arachnoid villi with the central aspect of the villi being continuous with the subarachnoid space. With trauma, acceleration-deceleration injury or traumatic injury the arachnoid villi are damaged. There is a danger of the development of a hygroma—dissection of the CSF into the arachnoid membrane since the CSF is under a pressure. The pia meter is the most intimate layer of all of the dural layers. This intimate relationship is maintained throughout the entirety of the central nervous system. It has been demonstrated histologically that the attachments are seen as flattened cells with long thin winding processes. As mentioned previously, the pia mater and the arachnoid are together collectively referred to as the leptomininges. The pia is separated from the surface of the brain by the glial basement membrane and the subpial space. Pial cells have a specific arrangement as well with single layers and then multiple layers. The pia intima is the closest layer of the pia to the brain matter and is made of single processes and a collagen cell. In areas where there are multiple layers, the tissue is defined as the epipial layer. Generally speaking, the pial is found to be thicker as it surrounds the spinal cord than that which surrounds the brain.

Small vessels will penetrate the brain surface and that of the spinal cord. Where this cellular arrangement is the case, there are small envelopes of pial cell processes that are found within the surface of the brain and spinal cord and these spaces are called perivascular spaces or Virchow-Robin spaces. This tissue has a very unique structure as well. From each ligament there extends a series of 20-30 shark like teeth structures. These structures are seen to extend laterally and will attach to the inner surface of the arachnoid lined dural sac. The second pial modification is the filum terminale. This is a tough strand of pial mater that extends caudally from the conus medularis and attaches the cord to the spinal column. This attachment is accomplished by the attachment of the dural sac and then the coccyx as the coccygeal ligament.

CHAPTER 11

CEREBROVASCULAR SYSTEM

The Cerebrovascular system of the brain is responsible for providing the nourishment of the brain as well as being a mechanism for the transport of signals within the blood for brain activity. The human brain accounts for only 2% of the total bodyweight of an adult human yet it accounts for more than 20% of the oxygen consumption and 17% of the total cardiac output. These numbers demonstrate a tremendous activity level of the brain. Approximately 50% of the problems associated with resultant neurologic deficit are due to a vascular origin. This includes the traditional cerebrovascular bleed and the transient ischemic attacks. The major cause of migraine headaches and cluster headaches are vascular in nature as well. Typically, an individual will experience loss of consciousness if the brain is deprived of oxygen in as short a period of time as 10-12 seconds. Brain injury is evident with oxygen deprivation of 3 to 5 minutes. This reflects the tremendous energy consumption of the brain. The discussion of the reduction of core body temperature after injury of cerebral bleed will not be discussed in this chapter but rather this is a pure review of the system and its function.

The brain derives its blood supply from a variety of vessels, the paired internal carotid arteries and the paired vertebral arteries. The arterial supplies from the internal carotid arteries will further subdivide into structures called the anterior and middle cerebral arteries. The opposite is true for the paired vertebral arteries as they will join to form the basilar artery. The basilar artery will travel along the surface of the brain and then it will bifurcate into the right and left posterior cerebral arteries.

The Internal Carotid artery is a product of three segments as it travels superiorly towards its entry into the skull. These distal segments are the petrous, cavernous and cerebral portions. The petrous portion is located within the carotid canal and has no identifiable branches. The cavernous part passes through the cavernous sinus and branches to become the hypophysial branch and the meningeal branch. The cerebral branch is unique in that is identified as soon as it penetrates the dura slightly ventral to the optic nerve. There are a number of branches that come from the cerebral branch, the ophthalmic, posterior communicating, and the anterior choroidal artery. The ophthalmic artery branches off to give rise to the central artery of the retina. The posterior communicating artery will join the posterior cerebral artery and the anterior choroidal artery as they travel along the optic tract. The internal carotid artery terminates as the anterior and middle cerebral arteries.

The anterior cerebral artery is a unique structure in that it acts as the beginning of a circuit of circulation that allows for the occlusion of one portion of the blood supply to be compensated for by the structure of the vasculature itself in a retro-circuit manner. This system is well known and understood and called the Circle of Willis. In this system, the anterior cerebral artery will ride on top of the optic chiasm where it will be joined by the other mirror image of the anterior cerebral artery. The specific portion of the anterior cerebral artery as it projects communicating artery is called the A1 segment. This is important since the anterior communicating artery and its distal segments lie within the cistern of the lamina terminalis. The anterior cerebral artery branches over the medial surface of the hemisphere to the level of the parieto-occipital sulcus and this aspect of the artery is termed the A2 segment, this is important because the terminal branches of the A2 segment lie within the callosal cistern.

The middle cerebral artery is more often larger than the other terminal branches. Anatomically, the portion of the vessel that lies from the origin of the internal carotid and the point where it will branch deep in the Sylvian Fissure is known as the M1 segment. Anatomically, this is important since the branches of this vessel are found to lie within the Sylvian cistern. The M1 segment will bifurcate as it courses over the ventromedial aspect of the insular cortex. The trunks that are seen to branch from the middle cerebral artery at this point are called the M2 segment. The branches of this aspect of the middle cerebral artery will provide circulation for the insular cortex.

The vertebral artery has a very unusual path as it traverses the upper cervical column and the base of the skull. It will exit the vertebral column at the transverse foramen of C1 pass caudally and then turn medially as it will pass the lateral aspect of the atlas. It is seen to penetrate the alanto-occipital membrane to which it has structural anchors. As the vertebral artery passes into the subarachnoid space, it will lie within the lateral cerebellomedullary cistern. There are many branches that project from this main vessel. The first branch is the posterior inferior cerebellar artery (PICA) with its perfusion of the dorsolateral medulla. The PICA is located within the cisterna magna and supplies the choroid plexus of the fourth ventricle. The next branch is less clear in the true origin as there are variations in the point of origin for the posterior spinal artery. In 25% of humans, the posterior spinal artery arises from the vertebral artery. The posterior spinal artery perfuses the area distal to the PICA on the same dorsolateral aspect of the medulla. This artery will move towards the midline and give rise to the anterior spinal artery that is found to lie within the premedullary cistern.

The Basilar artery is seen in the prepontine cistern. It also has many branches that it will give off. The first of these branches is the anterior inferior cerebellar artery (AICA). The AICA will follow the cerebellopontine cistern in its course through the brain caudal to the middle cerebellar peduncle. The anterior inferior cerebellar artery is responsible for perfusing the ventral and lateral aspects of the cerebellum, the pons, and the caudal aspect of the choroid plexus. There are branches off the AICA that will follow the course of the facial and vestibulocochlear nerve origins and follow them through the acoustic meatus called the labyrinthine artery. The third major branch of the basilar artery is the many pontine arteries that emanate from this artery. These arteries will themselves branch again and as they do so they will perfuse the pons as the paramedian arteries. There are two further subdivisions of these arteries, the short coursing short circumferential branches of the long circumferential branches. The last major branch of the basilar artery is the superior cerebellar artery. This artery is actually two arteries that perfuse the entire superior aspect of the cerebellum and the caudal aspects of the midbrain.

The posterior cerebral artery is a product of the bifurcation of the basilar artery as it lies within the interpeduncular cistern. The posterior cerebral artery is actually a paired set of arteries. The course of each individual branch will follow a path that goes just in front of the root of the occulomotor nerve. The perfusion of these branches will be the midbrain, thalamus, and the ventral and medial surfaces of the temporal and occipital lobes. Clarity of this branch is derived from the segmental division designated P1 thru P4. The initial segment is the P1 segment and it is found between the bifurcation of the basilar artery and the posterior communicating artery. The perfusion pattern of the P1 segment is completed by the terminal branches of the quadrigeminal and the thalamoperforating arteries. The next segment is the P2 segment and it is found between the posterior communicating artery and the inferior temporal branches. The perfusion pattern of this artery is completed by supply to the midbrain. The next segment to discuss will be the P3 segment that will provide terminating branches called the temporal branches. The last segment is the P4 segment. The P4 segment is responsible for the provision of the terminal calcerine artery and the parieto-occipital arteries.

As was previously mentioned, the circulatory system is quite unique system in the design with a redundant circulatory network called the Circle of Willis. The name does not belie the true shape of the structure as it has a hexagonal shape rather than a true circle. This structure is found on the ventral aspect of the brain and lies deep under the protection of the calverium floor. The brain has some very important anatomic structures that are found to lie within the structural aspect of the Circle of Willis. The optic chaism and the optic tracts, the infindibulium, the tuber cinereum, the hypothalamus, and the mamillary bodies are all contained within the Circle of Willis. There are deeper central branches that are given off by the Circle of Willis and these perforating arteries are subdivided into 4 groups. The anteriomedial group has its origins from the Anterior communicating artery and the A1 branch. The perforating arteries that arise from this aspect will provide circulation to the optic chaism and the anterior hypothalamus. The anterolateral group has origins from the M1 segment and will provide circulation to the **interior** aspects of the hemisphere.

CHAPTER 12

TELENCEPHALON

The largest and perhaps most conspicuous portion of the human brain is the telencephalon, or the cerebral hemispheres. The function of the cerebral corticies is higher cognitive functional behaviors, integration of sexual function, pain and emotional expression. Each hemisphere consists of the prototypic elevations and depressions that are pathoneumonic of the brain, the gyri and sulci. These are the recognizable elevations and depressions but the actual composition of the cerebral hemispheres are composed of an external layer of grey matter that sits over the inner white matter or cortex. These elevations and depressions are used as landmarks and therefore must show some amount of stability in their localization. There is however a variability that is seen as comparison of brain to brain is done. Overall, there is consistency in several of the elevations and depressions. Some neuroanatomists will discuss histological identification of slightly more than 200 subdivisions of brain tissue. The convolutions and elevations are seen throughout the brain, and they are seen to extend even from the lateral aspect into the separation of the hemispheres, the longitudinal cerebral fissure. The sulci and the gyri are used to define lobes of the brain as well as identify regions of function.

In order to understand these land marks the terms must be identified. A sulcus is a depression between gyri in the surface while the gyrus is the elevation or bump on the hemispheres. In the situation where the sulci are deep, they are then called fissures. On the lateral aspect of the brain, the central sulcus is one of the prominent invaginations. It divides the precentral gyrus from the postcentral gyrus. Medially, we can identify the calcarine sulcus, the collateral sulcus, the parietooccipital sulcus, and the cingulate sulcus. Laterally, we can define the precentral sulcus, postcentral sulcus, intraparietal sulcus, parietooccpital sulcus, superior frontal and the superior temporal sulcus. These main sulci are the major sulci used for identification and delineation of lobes and functional regions. The sulci and gyri known will be expanded upon further in this chapter. The telencephalic vessicles are differentiations from the primary vessicles. The proliferation of the ventral border zone tissue will eventually differentiate into the neuroblasts that will become the deep cortex tissue of the basal ganglia. The adult brain is well defined especially for the separation of the hemispheres. The dura will differentiate and leave the falx cerebri to separate the hemispheres. The primary vessicles upon completion of differentiation will produce six (6) anatomic lobes: Frontal, Parietal, Temporal, Occipital, Limbic, and Insular.

The frontal lobe is the largest of the lobes in the cerebral hemispheres, accounting for more than 1/3 of the total mass. The posterior border of the frontal lobe is the precentral gyrus. Therefore, everything anterior to the precentral gyrus is considered as frontal lobe. Anatomically, the most anterior of the frontal lobe mass is the prefrontal area. The frontal lobe is characterized by five (5) major gyri. These are the precentral gyrus, the superior, middle and inferior frontal lobe gyri, and the fronto-orbital gyrus. The frontal lobe is defined by the superior, middle and inferior frontal lobe gyri with a further subdivision of the inferior frontal gyri into the "pars" region. This mass of tissue runs at right angles to the precentral gyrus. The "pars" is composed of the pars opercularis, the pars orbitalis, and the pars triangularis. The mass of tissue seen to lie on the anterior aspect of the precentral gyrus will be the premotor area, while the tissue of the precentral gyrus is the primary motor cortex. The precentral gyrus is the larger one that runs parallel to the central sulcus.

The dominant hemisphere will contain Broca's area of speech expression. In a right handed person this dominant hemisphere will be the left cerebral hemisphere. Broca's area is located deep in the inferior frontal gyrus. We see the olfactory system comprising the main ventral portion of the frontal pole of the frontal lobe. The neural structure of the olfactory system is rather complex for one of the most archaic of senses. On the ventral surface of the frontal lobe are the olfactory bulbs. These projections of neural tissue are easily identifiable and run as a pair of long thin projections toward the anterior pole. They lie almost flat on the interior of the floor of the unforgiving skull. As they project posteriorly, they become identified as the olfactory tracts that lie between the orbital gyri. The termination point will be the anterior perforated substance. The olfactory tract runs within the olfactory sulcus that is identifiable as the lateral aspect of the gyrus rectus. As the olfactory tract moves posteriorly, the division of the fibers will form the trigone. This olfactory trigone is triangular shaped tissue that is composed of the medial and lateral olfactory striae with coverings from the remnants of the primitive cortical tissue. This tissue is defined as the medial and lateral olfactory gyri.

The parietal lobe has anatomic boarders that are defined by the central sulcus, the cingulate sulcus and the lateral fissure. The posterior border will be the line drawn from the parieto-occipital sulcus and the pre occipital notch. Within these confines will be the post central gyrus, the superior and inferior parietal lobes, the intraparietal sulcus, the supramarginal gyrus and the angular gyrus, the paracentral lobules (medially), and the preuncal cortex. The post central gyrus is found posterior to the central sulcus and almost parallel to the precentral gyrus. Functionally, this is the home of the somatosensory cortex. The superior and the inferior parietal lobes are found caudal to the precentral gyrus. The caudal portion of the paracentral lobule is the preuncal cortex and this mass is known to be involved in the functioning of the limbic lobe.

Deep within the cerebral hemispheres will be the Island of Reil or the insula. It is surrounded by the temporal, parietal and frontal lobes. The insula is another mass that serves in two systems as it is also considered as part of the limbic system. This is due to the rostrally located portion of the insula. Functionally we understand the insula to be involved in the integration of somatosensory input. It works in conjunction with the somatosensory cortex in the integration of those inputs. The reciprocal neural pathways are seen histologically.

The temporal lobe is found ventral to the lateral fissure. It is large and is covered by the temporal bone of the calvarium. Within the temporal lobe is the Transverse Gyrus of Heschl. This is an important land mark as it is within the temporal lobe that the majority of the auditory function is found. The occipitotemporal gyrus is found to be located on the ventral aspect of the lobe.

The occipital lobe is inclusive of the calcarine fissure and the visual cortex. This is the integration site for the visual system. It is found to occupy the most posterior aspect of the cortex.

Upon histologic examination of the tissue of the cerebral corticies, it becomes apparent that the distribution of the cell types is not uniform in its nature. The understanding of this variable distribution is that the distribution differences and the variability of the density of the cell distribution is based on functional characteristics of the tissue being examined. It has been well investigated and documented that the distribution of the cellular components of the cortices is arranged in a horizontal layered manner. Many authors describe the neuron designation as "belonging to the layer according to the position of the cell body". This definition of descriptive layering makes it easy to compartmentalize neurons. This is because of the numerical arrangement of the layers running from most superficial to the deepest. It is important to remember the terminology in neuroscience has the word "laminae" to be analogous to the word layer. Therefore layers of tissue are considered as laminae as well. In layer 1, the cells identified are those closest to the pia mater. It is generally free of neuronal cell bodies, however, it is strong it the apical dendrites of the pyramidal cells. This is a layer called the plexiform or the molecular layer. In this description of layers, layer 2 is seen to have a dense population of small pyramidal neuronal cell bodies. With staining, this layer has a granular appearance. Moving deeper, the third layer is densely packed with larger pyramidal cell bodies. Interestingly, the size of the cell body increases with depth. The next deeper layer is layer 4, and it is seen to contain the most densely packed array of cells in the cortical layers. The components of this layer are the small round cell bodies of the stellate cells and the haphazardly arranged pyramidal cell bodies. This layer demonstrates the unorganized arrangement and alignment of the pyramidal cell bodies that differentiates them from the previous layers. Layer 5 hold true to the theorem of increasing cell size with increasing depth as layer 5 is composed of the largest pyramidal cell bodies of all the layers. Conversely, the density of packing is least in this layer. Penetrating into the 6th layer of the cortex will be the most unusual arrayed neurons as it is composed of the multiform neuronal cell bodies.

In the corticies, information that is transmitted from the periphery to the termination pint will pass along or through the subcortical white matter. These fibers that constitute the underlying structures are myelinated. Unlike the organization of the laminae described above these fibers are arranges in bundles of association tracts that will produce interconnections between differing areas. It is possible that these associative tract fibers may even cross into the other hemispheres or just be connections of adjacent gyri. These fibers may be short association fibers or they may be long association fibers. The name implies general characteristics of the fibers and where they act as connections. It is possible that the fibers may be commisural bundles that specifically connect the right and left hemispheres and finally they may be fibers of the internal capsule. Experimental evidence has demonstrated that the superior longitudinal fasciculus will provide the connections for the frontal, occipital and parietal lobes. These are in contrast to the arcuate fasciculus that has been identified as the connection between the frontal and the temporal lobes. The fibers that are seen to connect the frontal and the occipital areas within the white myelinated fibers will be the inferior frontooccipital fasciculus. The commissural fibers are exemplified by the corpus callosum. This is the largest collection of commissural fibers and it demonstrates how these fibers are destined to connect corresponding structures. These structures are able to be in either hemisphere.

Anatomically, the corpus callosum fibers are seen in the roof of the lateral ventricle. The interconnections of this mass of tissue have subcatagorizations as have been demonstrated histologically. The frontal lobes are connected by the frontal or the minor forceps while the connections for the occipital lobe are via the major or the occipital forceps. Next, we identify the fibers that connect the tapetum that connects the remaining portion of the occipital lobes. These fibers are known to compose the main structure of the Genu, the rostrum, the splenum and the body. In some differing texts the body is described as the trunk. Other commissural fibers will be identified through the hippocampus as the hippocampal fibers, the anterior commissure fibers, the posterior commissure fibers and the habenular fibers. The hippocampal fibers are the interconnections for the frontal and temporal lobes. This will provide a multitude of connection paths. There are fibers crossing the midline that are seen to originate in the hippocampus and then traverse the fibers outside of the splenium of the corpus callosum as mentioned above. The habenular nuclei are connected via fibers within the dorsal posterior commissure.

The internal capsule is composed of projection fibers that have origins outside of the telencephalon but still within the cerebral cortex (corticopectal fibers—thalamocortical fibers) and those that have axonal origin within the cortex and project to areas outside (corticofugal fibers—corticospinal fibers).

The basal ganglia have undergone some intense investigation over the past 15 years as the interest in the motor disturbance portion of Parkinson's disease has gained more public awareness. The basal ganglia are collections of several differing subtypes of tissue. The primary functional responsibility of the basal ganglia is in the motor component of the nervous system. The dorsal basal ganglia that is composed of the caudate and the lenticular nuclei and the ventral basal ganglia composed of the nucleus accumbens and the olfactory tubercle. Lastly, the basal ganglia contain the ventral palladium that is itself composed of the substantia innominata. The substantia innominata is also known as the basal nucleus of Meynert and is found deep to the anterior perforated substance. It is millimeters outside the fibers of the anterior commissure. Histological examination of those individuals diagnosed with Alzheimer's Disease demonstrate significant alterations in the homogeneity of the cells that compose this tissue mass.

It is an unusual arrangement to have the olfactory tubercle as a portion of the basal ganglia, however the understanding of the embryologic development will make this more understandable. The corpus striatum is composed of the lenticular nuclei and the caudate. This is important as one of the surgical treatments for Parkinson's disease is directly related to one of the aspects of this structure. The globus pallidum is a surgical target to resolve some of the symptoms of Parkinson's Disease. The globus pallidus is a subdivision of the corpus striatum, as it is subdivided into the neostriatum (caudate nucleus and the putamen) and the paleostraium (the globus pallidus). The caudate nucleus, the head, tail and body, is found on the lateral ventricle wall. The head of the caudate is evidenced as a bump on the anterior horn and from that point the body will project caudally to become the body. The tail of the caudate changes position as it will project slightly ventrally and anteriorly. The lenticular nucleus is composed of the globus pallidus and the putamen and is found surrounded by white matter at the base of the hemisphere. The globus pallidus is found slightly deeper than the putamen with an internal and external component. The globus pallidum is afforded isolation for the surgical ablation from the putamen by the thin layer of the lamina white matter. The globus pallidum is slightly smaller than the putamen in mass as well as being located deeper. Although not anatomically a component of the telencephalon, the substantia nigra (midbrain) and the subthalamic nucleus (diencephalon) functionally are intimately intertwined with the role of the basal ganglia. The substantia nigra is located caudal to the subthalamic nuclei and dorsomedial to the crus cerebri and subdivided into the pars reticulata and the pars compacta. The pars compacta is identified by the large numbers neuronal cell bodies increased content of melanin. The function of the basal ganglia is to be a relay center for the brain. The lenticular fascicule is one of these connection bundles of neuron that have been identified. Fibers of the lenticular fasciculus will project through the internal capsule from the globus pallidus. These delicate connections will become the thalamic fasciculi and this is how the intimate relationship between the thalamic nuclei and the higher centers of the brain become intertwined. The anterior aspect of the internal capsule sends projections to the thalamic fasciculus. These fibers will join in the fibers from the lenticular fasciculus as they then enter the thalamic fasciculus. This is unlike the fibers directly originating from the lenticular fasciculus as they have origins in the posterior internal capsule. The substantia nigra is connected to the neostriatum by the nigrostriatial projections while those that connect the striatum and the substantia nigra are the striatianigral projections. These are fine but important projection fibers as these connections are important in the manner they pass through the internal capsule.

The hippocampus is called the hippocampal formation since it is contains three (3) components, the dentate gyrus, the hippocampus and the subiculum. Anatomically, the parahippocampal gyrus is found within the subiculum. Projections of larger bundles of fibers from this hippocampal formation are the fibers of the fornix. The fornix can be further subdivided into the body, the crus, and the fimbria. The fimbria fibers will project along the dentate gyrus and the fibers of the crus. These fibers of the fornix are the main efferent projections from the hippocampus. Adjacent to the hippocampal formation will be the amygdala. This is a structure that is also composed of a variety of subunits of tissue. The ventral amygdalofugal bundle is one of the efferent projections from the amygdala and the other main efferent projection is the stria terminalis. The projections from the stria terminalis will continue on to the hypothalamus, the neostriatum and the septal tissue, while those of the ventral amygdalofugal projections will pass to the hypothalamus and the septum, but will also project to some areas of the brainstem. These connections are important because of the connections of the septal nuclei with the hippocampus, the amygdala and the limbic tissue. The manner these structures are so inter-related demonstrates the delicate line of catastrophic injury versus one that may be of slight in presentation. It also clearly demonstrates the need for a clear understanding of the structures and the function associated to them not only for diagnostic accuracy but also for a clear understanding of the clinical outcome.

CHAPTER 13

DIENCEPHALON

In the developing nervous system the developing cerebral hemispheres are considered the diencephalon. The swellings of the embryo are apparent in the human embryo as it nears 12 mm. It is at this time the thalamus, hypothalamus, epithalamus and subthalamus become distinguishable. The pace of the growth at this point is incredibly rapid. Within the human brain there are landmarks that we utilize for the identification of aspects of the brain. The demarcation of the midbrain from the diencephalon is found to be an imaginary line running from the posterior commissure and extending to the caudal aspect of the Mamillary body. This is the internal delineation, while the ventral or outer demarcation is found to follow the optic tract. In the development of the diencephalon, the initial point is the development is the hypothalamic groove as it is found on the wall of the third ventricle. This is important as it is the dividing line for the alar plate into the dorsal and ventral portions. These two tissue masses with further differentiate into the dorsal thalamus (thalamus) and the hypothalamus. The mass of the dorsal thalamus will continue to differentiate into the interthalamic adhesion. The differentiation of the roof of the third ventricle will produce the pineal gland and rostrally, the habenular nuclei. Interconnected with the development of the cerebral hemispheres will be the pituitary gland as it will differentiate from the floor of the third ventricle as the joining of the infundibulum (the posterior pituitary lobe) and Rathke's pouch. This joining of the tissue is important as the anterior lobe of the pituitary gland (adenohypophysis) and the pars intermedia will be produced. Located between the thalamic nuclei and the hypothalamus will be the third ventricle. The differentiation is important as the structures that will be produced include the pineal gland and the thalamic nuclei.

The diencephalon houses a large reservoir of cerebral spinal fluid within the third ventricle. This ventricle is found to occupy a midline position between the large dorsal thalamus and the hypothalamus. The diencephalon is composed of the thalamus and its subdivisions and the fibers of the internal capsule. At first glance this does not appear to be of much significance because of the comparatively low numbers of structures in the initial divisions, however, the function of the tissue represented and the compactness of the neurons quickly dispels that theory. The thalamus is considered as the great relay center of the brain. There is not much activity of the brain that does not either project through the thalamus or have reciprocal paths from the thalamus. The thalamus is actively engaged in influencing activity of the sensory, motor, and limbic systems. The thalamus is composed of subdivisions of neurons that will make up the dorsal thalamus, the ventral thalamus and the epithalamus. Each of these structures will see multiple subdivisions of neurons as well.

The lateral aspect of the dorsal thalamus is covered by the external medullary lamina (lamina—layer or sheet of tissue) consisting of myelinated fibers. The fibers of this white matter contain the neurons of the thalamic reticular nucleus. Additional myelination is seen in the internal medullary lamina. The internal medullary lamina is a very important structure anatomically, as it provides the separation of the thalamus. It is shown to plunge into the core of the thalamus as it provides this separation of the anterior, lateral, medial and intralaminar nuclei. The anterior thalamic nuclei are composed of a composite of smaller nuclei, the anterior nucleus of the thalamus. The position it occupies in the thalamus will produce a eminence that will be the anterior thalamic tubercle. Projection neurons from this tubercle will pass through the internal capsule anteriorly and continue on to the cingulate gyrus. The dorsomedial nuclei are also composed of multiple subdivisions of neurons. The parvocellular, the magnocellular and the internal medullary lamina collectively will form the dorsomedial nuclei of the thalamus. Functionally, the connections of these subdivisions are the temporal and frontal lobe and the substantia nigra. The former are from the parvocellular and the magnocellular nuclei and the latter projects from the substantia nigra and some from the frontal lobe as well. Anatomically, the former are larger than the latter. The larger of the subdivisions is the lateral thalamic nuclei. As it is larger, it has many subdivisions within it. These subdivisions are grouped in structural aggregates called "tiers". The dorsal tier is further subdivided into the lateral dorsal thalamic nuclei and the lateral posterior nuclei. The pulvinar nucleus is also subdivided further as the anterior, medial, lateral, and the inferior nuclei. Collectively, these nuclei subdivisions are found functionally related to the motor control of the eyes and the visual integration. This is evidenced by the connection with the superior colliculus, the visual association cortex (inferior) the temporal, parietal and frontal lobes (medial, lateral, anterior). The ventral tier is composed of the ventral anterior nucleus, the ventral lateral nucleus, the ventral posteriolateral, and the ventral posteriomedial nuclei. Collectively the inputs are from the motor and the somatosensory systems. The ventral lateral and the ventral anterior are the motor aspects while the ventral posterolateral and the ventral posteriomedial are the somatosensory aspects. The ventral lateral nucleus is further subdivided into the pars oralis, the pars medialis and the pars caudalis. The connections with the globus pallidus, the cerebellum, and the frontal lobe show the multitude of connections that are influenced by the ventral nucleus and the thalamus as a whole. The ventral posterior inferior nucleus will receive projections from the vestibular relay on their way to the deep central sulcus at the postcentral gyrus. The ventral intermediate nucleus is seen to have connections from the cerebellum and then project on the frontal lobe. The ventral posteriomedial nucleus has projections to it from the trigeminothalamic, the spinal trigeminal and the principle trigeminal sensory nucleus. The ventral posteriormedial nucleus will receive projections from the spinothalamic fibers of the cord. This is another demonstration of a collectively compacted set of neurons that if pathologically impacted will demonstrate catastrophic effects.

The suprageniculate nucleus, the nucleus limitians, and the posterior nucleus will constitute the posterior nucleus complex proper. This is a pain sensation complex, (nocioception) that will project on to the cortex via the somatosensory pathways. The intralaminar nuclei show neural projections into the cortex, the striatum and additional thalamic nuclei. The centromedian mass projects to the motor areas of the cerebral cortex and the striatum while the parafascicular nuclei projects to the frontal lobe rostrally and laterally. In an unusual twist, the thalamic reticular nucleus projections to it come from the cortex while it shows none in reciprocation with the cortex; however it demonstrates a series of projection back into itself. Functionally this is a mass of neurons whose activity is in the modulation of the impulses that pass through it and not as a direct conduit. The projections into it are seen to originate in the thalamocortical and the corticothalamic paths. The midline thalamic nuclei are seen to show projections to the dorsal thalamus and the reticular nucleus. These neurons show projections into the amygdyla and the cingulate cortex. The midline thalamic nuclei have experimental evidence that they functionally are active in the visceral activities of the body.

The hypothalamus is best known as the thermoregulatory center of the brain. It is related to the functional activity of the limbic lobe and as such these thermoregulatory controls make perfect sense. However, the additional activity in the visceromotor, viscerosensory and endocrine systems will be considered here as well. As the hypothalamus is the main regulator of the autonomic nervous system, and the viscerosensory "gauge' (blood pH, hormone levels etc), its functional control mechanisms on the anterior pituitary, and its effects on the production and release of oxytocin and vasopressin, it is easy to comprehend how it can imply regulatory effects across these many tissues. Structurally, the hypothalamus is able to be divided into periventricular, lateral and medial zones. The periventricular zone consists of the neurons bordering the ependymal aspect of the lateral ventricle. The position is occupies is belied by the name "periventricular" zone. The lateral zone is demonstrated histologically to run the length of the hypothalamus. This mass of tissue carries a very important functional responsibility as it is imperative for the cardiovascular function and in satiety. The medial zone is seen to contain (3) subdivisions. These subdivisions are the tuberal, mamillary and the chiasmatic regions. The chaismatic region is further subdivided into (5) five regions: the anterior, the preoptic, the supraoptic, paraventricular, and the suprachaismatic regions. These regions are important as they have regulatory effects on the cardiovascular functioning via the anterior, the hormone release via the preoptic-supraoptic-periventricular regions, the regulation of body thermodynamic activity via the preoptic regions. Therefore, damage to these areas can have global implications. The human satiety center is located within the ventromedial nucleus. The functional aspect of the ventromedial nucleus is the release of proteins from the arcuate nucleus into the portal blood circulation to move to the anterior pituitary. Biochemically, these are inhibiting factors and others are stimulating factors. The mammillary nuclei and the posterior nucleus compose the bulk of the mass of the mammillary region. Functionally, the mammillary nuclei are involved in the formation of memory traces and the feeding activities. The posterior nucleus is involved with the increases in blood pressure, the act of shivering and pupillary dilation. The communication with the mammillary nuclei and the posterior nuclei with the fornix demonstrates the intimate relationship between the thalamic nuclei and the more rostral aspects of the nervous system.

There are many afferent communication pathways known to be present, the fornix fibers that have origins in the hippocampus and the stria terminalis whose fibers have origins in the amygdyla along with those of the ventral amygdalofugal bundle and those of the medial forebrain bundle are thalamic nuclei of importance.

The pineal gland, the habenular nuclei and the stria medullaris are collectively known as the epithalamus. The pineal is unique in that it does not contain neurons, and still maintains implications in the ability to sense light. The pinelocytes are designed for the manufacturing of melatonin and serotonin. In the course of the biochemical activity of the nervous system as it relates to other physiologic functions, these cells are responsible for the sleep cycle as it is related to the exposure of light. Exposure of light will diminish the release of the serotonin N acetyltransferase, and the production of melatonin. Therefore, it is necessary for the human body to experience dampened light sources for the increased activity of these enzymes. It is a very unusual mechanism of action that the pinealocyte exerts its effect as it is a secondary effect. The preganglionic sympathetic neurons will project to the superior cervical ganglion that will synapse on the postganglionic fibers riding on the internal carotid to the pineal gland. It is the sequence of transmission that produces the mechanism of action for the photo effect for the pineal gland and the circadium rhythm. The importance from a biochemical aspect, of these pinealocytes is not limited to the effect of the manufacturing of melatonin, but also the production of serotonin, thyrotropin releasing hormone and norepinepherine. Interestingly, these substances are available for release in the circulation or the cerebrospinal fluid. The relationship with the habenular nuclei is seen with the direct anatomic position of the habenular nuclei as they sit anterior to the pineal gland. The habenular nuclei is actually composed of two (2) masses of tissue, the lateral and the medial nucleus. Of the two, the lateral is the larger and together, they form the habenulo-interpeduncular tract (fasciculus retroflexus) that terminates in the interpeduncular nucleus of the midbrain. The stria medullaris thalami is seen to lay over the dorsal aspect of the thalamus and it receives inputs from the medial and the lateral habenular nuclei. The entire mass of tissue is connected together via the habenular commissure.

The subthalamus is also known as the ventral thalamus. As was discussed previously, the ventral thalamus is the smallest aspect of the diencephalon. The size of the tissue mass is not in correlation to its importance however. This mass of tissue includes the field of Forel (the prerubral area) and the zona incerta. The subthalamic nucleus is located as a “lens shaped” rostral and dorsal to the substantia nigra and ventral to the lenticular fasciculus. The importance of these cells is in the inputs that they receive as inputs are from the motor areas of the cerebral cortex with parallel reciprocal connection to the globus pallidus. The zona incerta is found to be located dorsally in relation to the subthalamic nuclei. These fibers are important as they are the outputs for the pons, the pretectal, cerebral cortex and the colliculi. There are also fibers from the prerubral area (Forel's Field) that are subdivided into the $H_1$and the H_2 areas that are projections from the thalamic nuclei. More specifically, we see the fibers projecting from the lenticular fasciculus representing H1 that will project into those cells that make up the mass of the myelinated fibers of the thalamic fasciculus representing H2. This mass of tissue is particularly susceptible to vascular types of injury or hyoperfusion types of pathologic insult. These types of insults will elicit hemiballismus. This is seen to manifest itself contralaterally.

CHAPTER 14

MIDBRAIN

This is the smallest mass of the brain as measured by shear mass. However, the mass of the midbrain does not convey the importance it has for the overall system. There are many landmarks that are utilized on the dorsal surface of the midbrain and many structures that are known to emerge that signify the importance of the mass. The midbrain is extensively organized internally as we identify the cerebral aqueduct, the periaqueductal grey matter, the tegmentum, the red nucleus, the substantia nigra, and occulomotor complex. Inspection of the transverse section of the mid brain will be defined by the superior and the inferior colliculi. The structural components as mentioned above include the periaqueductal grey matter. This is important as these cells are densely packed surrounding the cerebral aqueduct. Histologically, the subdivisions of the periaqueductal grey matter will be defined by the types of histochemical properties they exhibit. There is a variety of substances that are demonstrated here, serotonin, enkephalin, endorphins, and other neuropeptides as well. There is much experimental evidence to suggest that the periaqueductal gray matter is involved in the brains interpretation of pain. Projections to the raph magnus and the paragigantocellular nucleus of the reticular formation will continue on to the spinothalamic tract.

The substantia nigra is found within the rostral portion of the midbrain. It is found to lie adjacent to the crus cerebri. The structural components of the substantia nigra are the pars reticulata and the pars compacta. The reticulata is situated ventrally, while the compacta is found to lie dorsally. The reticulata sends very small projection neurons to the thalamus and the superior colliculus. The pathoneumonic aspect of the substantia nigra is the use of dopamine as the main neurotransmitter. Histologic staining reveals that the darkened dopaminergic neurons project almost entirely to the basal ganglia. This is the basis for the pathologic syndrome associated to Parkinson's disease, a degeneration of the neurons utilizing the dopamine neurotransmitter. The basal ganglia or more correctly, the basal nuclei, are a set of paralleled neural circuits that connect the cerebral cortex to the thalamus, running through the basal ganglia. This paralleled neural circuitry gives rise to a multitude of problems with damage to the area. It is clear to understand the implications to the motor pathways with damage, but damage is not limited to just motor paths. There is associated damage in the ability to interpret data, thought processing is disrupted, and so is the ability to perceive things in the environment. The basal ganglia are a very complex array of neurons. Typical division of the basal ganglia will look like this: a dorsal division and a ventral division. The dorsal division will include the caudate, putamen, substantia nigra, subthalamic nuclei, and the parabrachial pontine reticular formation while the ventral division will include the globus pallidus, substantia innominata, nucleus basalis of Meynert, the olfactory tubercle and the nucleus accumbens. The components of the basal ganglia and the interactions with the higher levels and the lower spinal centers are a complex series of interactions and interrelations. The striatal complex is subdivided into the neostriatum (caudate nucleus, putamen) and the ventral striatum (nucleus accumbens, olfactory tubercle). The caudate nucleus and the putamen have like origins but are kept apart by the fibers of the internal capsule. The striatal complex is defined by a specific set of tissue the striasomes, which neurons lacking in acetylcholinesterase and increased numbers of opioid receptors. Further histologic investigation will reveal large amounts of neuropeptide activity in these neurons. These are most evident in the head of the caudate. Histologically, this is in direct contrast to the remainder of the caudate, the matrix, which contains large amounts of acetylcholinesterase. This will allow demonstration of the differences in the tissue under stain and it will elucidate the neuronal pathways from the cerebral cortex to the striatum, the corticostriatial paths. These are afferent pathways and provide inputs just like those from the thalamus, thalamostriatial fibers, the substantia nigra (nigrostiatal fibers), and the parabrachial pontine reticular fibers. The efferent projections will proceed to the pallidum as the striatopallidal fibers. There will be a small amount of projections that will run on to the thalamus and some to the nigral complex as the striatonigral fibers. Neurons associated with the striatum are called medium spiny neurons. Structurally, they are extensively arborized and very limited receptive fields. Because of the limited receptive field, the inputs are limited to the strisome in which the cell body is located. Characteristic neurotransmitter for these medium spiny neurons is a series of inhibitory neurotransmitters such as GABA. These medium spiny neurons are also capable of producing a modulatory effect through the capacity to use neuroactive peptides. Clinically, Huntington's Disease is a direct representation of the loss of the medium spiny neurons within the straitum.

The inhibitory neurotransmitter GABA is associated with the ventral pallidum as it is a tonic inhibitor of its target tissue. The globus pallidus is a mass of tissue that is subdivided into (2) two segments, the medial and the lateral segments. The medial segment is considered as the primary efferent projection of the basal ganglia. Each of the segments is inter-related via pallidopallidal fibers. The ventral pallidum is intimately associated with the substantia innominata, a mass of tissue that is found ventral to the anterior commissure and deep to the anterior perforated substance. The medial segment of the globus pallidus sends projections to the thalamus as the pallidothalamic fibers. This is termed the direct basal ganglia pathway. Upon exiting the globus pallidus, the fibers will project either as the ansa lenticularis or as the lenticular fasciculus. Though both fiber bundles have somewhat common origins, the projections are distinctly different. The ansa lenticularis has been identified to originate in the lateral aspect of the medial segment. This fiber will project on to the posterior limb of the internal capsule and on into the H field of Forel from the internal capsule. The lenticular fasciculus has been demonstrated to have its origins in the dorsomedial aspect of the medial segment. These fibers will also project through the internal capsule as they adjoin to produce the lenticular fasciculus. These fibers will also project on to the H field of Forel to join with the ansa lenticularis producing the thalamic fasciculus. The thalamic fasciculus will ride dorsal to the zona incerta to project on to the ventral lateral, the ventral anterior, and the centromedian nuclei of the thalamus. As mentioned above, the basal nucleus of Meynert is a special set of neurons that contain large amounts of acetylcholine. This is evidenced by the histologic staining of the neurons. Damage to this collection of neurons will produce Alzeheimer's disease. The lateral division of the globus pallidus is made up of the external or lateral segment and the ventral pallidum. The lateral division is also called the indirect pathway. It is called the indirect pathway as the inputs from the striatopallidal fibers, the substantia nigra pars reticularis and the subthalamopallital fibers will project to the subthalamic nucleus as the pallidosubthalamic fibers) and the substantia nigra as the pallidonigral fibers.

There is a very significant mass of corticofugal neurons that are seen to project to the internal capsule and then on to the brainstem and or spinal cord.

CHAPTER 15

BRAIN STEM

The Brainstem is composed of the medulla, the pons and the midbrain or in other words, the mesencephalon and the rhombencephalon without the cerebellum.

The medulla is found at the level of the foramen magnum. It is this landmark where the spinal cord merges with the most caudal aspect of the brain. This point of merger is the myelencephalon or the medulla oblongata. There is a structure associated with this joining of tissue, the pyramidal mass. There are many important structures associated with the compacted tissue within this area. Mainly, the cranial nerves are seen to exit the ventral side of the brain. The cranial nerves expected to be identified in this area will be CN 6(abducens), CN 7 (facial), CN 8 (vestibulocochlear), CN 9 (glossopharyngeal), CN 10 (vagus), CN 11 (accessory), and CN 12 (hypoglossal). Collectively these are referred to as the pons-medulla junctional cranial nerves.

Development of the brainstem is from the inferior aspect of the neural tube with the developing alterations in tissue configuration. Each of the neural tube configuration changes are of prime importance as the changes in direction demonstrate the eventual cervical and cephalic flexures. Continued development will produce the expansion of the central canal into the pyramidal shaped structure seen in the adult brain. This central canal will differentiate into the cerebral aqueduct of the adult brain. The significance of this structure will be evident as it passes through the tegmentum, the cereberal peduncles and finally the quadrigeminal plate.

Externally, the structural characteristics of the brainstem are the myelencephalon (medulla), the metencephalon (Pons) and the mesencephalon (midbrain). Internally, the brainstem is seen to consist of the tectum, the tegmentum and the basis. The pons is seen on the ventral aspect of the brainstem or the metencephalon. One must understand the structures from a both a structural and developmental aspect. The cerebellum is a part of the metencephalon, however it is not considered as a component of the functional part of the brainstem. The pons is a very bulbous projection from the ventral surface and it is the typical presentation from a sagittal viewing of the brain that is the most identifying view. In conjunction with this view will be the open voids seen in the brain stem that are the ventricles. These are the voids containing the cerebrospinal fluid. The system is a multiple set of openings and compartments. Within this system of openings and connections are the cerebral aqueduct (void of choroid plexus), the fourth ventricle, the foramen of Magendi, the cistern magna (dorsal cerebromedullary cistern), the paired foramen of Luschka, and the lateral recesses. Structurally, the cerebral aqueduct is found within the mesencephalon while the fourth ventricle is found within the rhombencephalon. The floor of the fourth ventricle is the rhomboid fossa. The roof of the fourth ventricle is produced by the anterior medullary velum (rostral) and the tela chordia(caudally). The walls of the fourth ventricle are found to be from the superior cerebellar peduncles, the middle and the inferior peduncles. There are a variety of identifying elevations in the floor of the rhomboid fossa for several cranial nerves. The rhomboid fossa is divided by the median sulcus and each half is quartered by the sulcus limitians. The fourth ventricle is connected to the third ventricle by the cerebral aqueduct. The fourth ventricle is also communicating with the central canal of the spinal cord at its caudal most point. Additional to the rostral and caudal opening are the three openings that allow the flow of CSF into the subarachnoid space. These three openings are the foramen of Magendi that lies in the midline and the paired lateral foramen of Luschka. These openings of the foramen of Luschka are seen at the ends of the lateral recesses of the fourth ventricle and open into the subarachnoid space via the cerebellopontine angles. The foramen of Magendi opens into the dorsal cerebromedullary cistern or the cistern magna. The lateral recesses of the system are found to wrap around the brainstem. The floor of the fourth ventricle is an important landmark that has within it the sulcus limitans, a depression located on the floor of the ventricle. The clinical importance of this groove is that it demonstrates the locale of the underlying cranial nerve tissue totality of the floor of the ventricle is called the rhomboid fossa that is known to be equally divided into the right and left halves by the median sulcus. Identification of this landmark is important in defining the functional characteristics of the underlying cranial nerve tissue as being either motor or sensory. Those nuclei found to lie between the sulcus limitans and the medial sulcus are functionally motor nerves. The facial colliculus is found within the medial aspect of the area between the sulcus limitans and the medial sulcus. Those cranial nerves located lateral to the sulcus limitans are sensory in function. Additionally, the vestibular area is located lateral to the sulcus limitans as well and is found to contain the vestibular nuclei.

The cerebellar peduncles are a component of the brainstem as was mentioned earlier in the chapter. There are three pairs of peduncles that constitute the connection with the cerebellum. Dorsally, there are zones of tissue called hillocks that are visualized. These zones are collectively called the corpora quadrigemina. There are 4 hillocks that will form this collection of tissue; these are the 2 superior colliculi and the 2 inferior colliculi. The importance of the brain stem is vast as it is known to influence many if not all cranial nerve nuclei, the flow of the CSF, the cerebellar peduncles, the reticular formation, monoaminergic neuronal paths, and both ascending as well as descending tracts.

Pathways through the Brainstem

Descending	**Ascending**
Corticospinal	Medial leminiscus
Corticonuclear	Spinothalamic
Central Trigeminal	Trigeminal leminiscus
Reticulospinal	Lateral Leminiscus
Corticopontine	Medial Longitudinal fasciculus
Rubrospinal	Inferior cerebellar peduncle
Tectospinal	Reticular formation
Medial Longitudinal Fasciculus	Superior cerebellar peduncle
Descending Trigeminal	Secondary vestibular
	Secondary gustatory

In the understanding of the brainstem, an in depth understanding of the brainstem nuclei is imperative. As the brainstem will develop, there are going to be differing basal plate components that will produce adult structures. There is alar plate origin for the sensory aspects of the brain stem nuclei. The nuclei subtypes present in adult life are the General somatic efferent, the Branchial efferents, and the General visceral efferents. These will be referred to by the abbreviations SE or GSE for the General Somatic Efferent, the SVE /BE representing the Special Visceral Efferents or the Branchial Efferents and the GVE or VE for the General Visceral Efferent nuclei. The GVE are found to be of parasympathetic preganglionic segment that will autonomically innervate the smooth muscles and the glands of the head—neck—torso, the Edinger-Westphal nucleus, the Superior & Inferior salivatory nucleus and lastly, the dorsal motor nucleus of the Vagus NN. The GSE or the General Somatic Efferents are known to innervate the somite origin striated muscles of the eyes and the tongue. Additionally, there is innervation to the hypoglossal, abducens, occulomotor and trochlear nuclei. The SVE /BE nuclei are known to innervate the muscles of mastication and swallowing, vocalizations, rotation of the head, and facial expression muscles. These muscles differ in origin as they originate from the branchial arches and not the somites. They are also known to innervate the facial NN nuclei, the spinal accessory nuclei, the V3 component of the facial NN and the nucleus ambiguous.

The sensory aspect of the brainstem nuclei originates from the General Somatic Afferents or the GSA, the General Visceral Afferent or the GVA and the Special Sense Nuclei. The GVA is responsible for the stimuli from the viscera and the tongue—epiglottis complex. There is also input from the solitary nucleus and the gustatory nucleus.

Cranial Nerves and Associated Nuclei

NAME	NERVE	NUCLEI
Occulomotor	CN III	Edinger—Westphal, Occulomotor
Trochlear	CN IV	Trochlear
Trigeminal	CN V	Descending Spinal NN, Mastication
Abducens	CN VI	Abducens
Facial	CN VII	Superior Salivatory Gustatory, facial
Vestibulocochlear	CN VIII	Cochlear—Vestibular
Glossopharyngeal	CN IX	Inferior Salivatory Nucleus Ambiguous
Vagas	CN X	Dorsal motor, nucleus ambigious
Accessory	CN XI	Spinal Accessory (C1-5)
Hypoglossal	CN XII	Hypoglossal

CHAPTER 16

MEDULLA

The medulla oblongata is also known as the myelencephalon. Anatomically, this is the most caudal portion of the brain. It is seen to extend from the foramen magnum to the level of the pons. The medulla presents with a cavity that is the continuation of the forth ventricle. It is not a large part of the overall mass of the brain as it comprises only 0.5% of the total mass. The importance of the structure is seen by the components that traverse it and the regulatory control it exerts. All the tracts that pass to the spinal cord to the brain and vise versa will pass through the medulla. Included in these components are 7 of the 12 cranial nerves. There is additional evidence of the importance of the medulla as it is the center of the cell groups that control both respiration and heart rate.

The developments of the basal plate that will give rise to the cells that differentiate into the hypoglossal nucleus are derived from the neuroblasts within the basal plate itself. Likewise, the cells that will differentiate to the nucleus ambiguous, the dorsal motor vagal nucleus and the inferior salivatory nucleus are from the same neuroblasts. The cells of the alar plate will differentiate into the cranial nerve nuclei, the vestibular nuclei, the cochlear nuclei, solitary nucleus, and the spinal trigeminal nucleus collectively. The alar neuroblast cells will differentiate in additional neurologic structures inferior to the obex as the inferior olivary complex. During the differentiation of these cells there will be seen differentiation of the neuroblastic cells that will become the pyramids.

Ventrally, the medulla has anatomic structures that are definitive for landmarks. The anterior or ventral medial fissure and adjacent elevations, the pyramids and the inferior olivary eminence are these landmarks. Within the pyramids are the fibers of decussation, the pyramidal decussation. It is within these confines of tissue that 90% of the fibers will cross over the midline. This collection of tissue is also referred to as the motor decussation. Within the borders of the medulla the rootlets of cranial nerve XII will exit within the confines of the preolivary sulcus. This shallow depression is found to lie between the pyramid and the olive. Along side the rootlets of CN XII, the hypoglossal, will run the fibers of cranial nerve IV, the Abducens nerve.

Inspection of the lateral aspect of the medulla elicits the postolivary sulcus, shallow channel running from the restiform body and the inferior olivary nucleus. The postolivary nucleus is the exit point of a variety of structures. Cranial nerves IX, glossopharyngeal, X, the Vagus and Cranial nerve XI, the Accessory nerve all exit from the postolivary nucleus. Looking at the dorsal surface of the medulla will yield the exit of the Cranial nerve VII, the facial and Cranial nerve VIII and the vestibulocochlear nerve. There is also a collection of nerve tissue that will form the trigeminal tubercle as they traverse the lateral aspect of the lateral medulla.

Dorsal inspection of the brain will yield structures that are important in the overall function of the medulla. The gracile fasciculi and the cuneate fasciculi are found to lie on the dorsal aspect of the medulla. They are however caudal to the obex. The restiform body is found to be rostral and lateral to the gracile and the cuneate. This is important as the fibers of the restiform body will join the smaller bundles of the juxtarestiform body and the resultant structure is the well defined inferior cerebellar peduncle.

The vasculature of the entire medulla and the choroid plexus of the 4th ventricle will be from the vertebral arteries. Specific branches of the vascular provision will be the anterior spinal artery to the medial aspect of the medulla, the vertebral artery to the ventrolateral medulla. The posterior inferior cerebellar artery will supply the dorsolateral medulla and finally the posterior spinal artery is the supply of the dorsal medulla.

The configuration of the brain and the spine has layers or sheets of tissue that provide a coordinated function. The ascending tracts of the nervous system will have originations from the spinal cord. These origins are not all the same for each ascending tract. In the tracts that make up the ascending path called the anterolateral system the origination is in the spinal cord gray matter. The anteriolateral system is comprised of the dorsal and ventral spinocerebellar tracts. Included in this bundle of nerve tissue are the fibers of the dorsal root ganglia. These fibers will also have differing destinations. There are some fibers that terminate as the spinoreticular fibers while others will proceed on to the thalamus. Dorsal column fibers will synapse within the medulla but there are fibers in this column that will also continue on as the medial lemniscal pathway. These fibers of the spinocerebellar tract will enter the cerebellum through the restiform body or through the superior cerebellar peduncle. There are additional fibers that have termination within the medulla, the spino-olivary and the spinovestibular fibers are some examples.

Just as there are tracts that ascend through the medulla or terminate in the medulla, there are fibers that originate in the medulla as descending tracts. The tracts that only traverse are those originating in the cerebral cortex, the corticospinal, the midbrain, rubrospinal-tectobulbospinal and the pons, the reticulospinal-vestibulospinal pathways. The paths that originate in the pons, the reticulospinal and the vestibulospinal tracts are unique in that there are additional fibers contributed to the pathways as they traverse the medulla.

The transition of the fibers from the medulla to the spinal cord is the aspect of the system that presents difficulty for most students. This fiber transition begins with the pyramidal decussation. It is here that the spinal cord gray matter will become the pyramidal decussation. The joining of the dorsolateral fasciculus and the substantia gelatinosa to form the spinal trigeminal tract is the landmark of the beginning of the medulla. The level of the most caudal medulla will see 90% of the corticospinal fibers cross the ventral midline. This crossing is at the level of the motor decussation or pyramidal decussation. The crossing of the fibers will form the contralateral corticospinal tract of the spinal cord. On the dorsal aspect of the medulla, the gracile and the cuneate fasiculi will merge to become the dorsal column. On the lateral aspect is the spinal trigeminal tract that will be superficial to the spinal trigeminal nucleus and the pars caudalis. This spinal trigeminal tract is made up of sensory fibers that will penetrate the brain as the trigeminal nerve and terminate on the spinal trigeminal nucleus. Additional projection of fibers from this nucleus will continue on to the contralateral thalamus as the ventral trigeminothalamic tract.

Laterally in the medulla, the ALS and the rubrospinal tract are deep to the dorsal and ventral spinocerebellar tract. The fibers of the ALS convey the pain and temperature input from the contralateral aspect of the body. Spinal trigeminal fibers carry the impulses from the ipsilateral side of the face. The ventral medulla is seen to carry the most rostral aspect of the accessory nucleus of cranial nerve XI as well as the remnants of the medial motor column, the medial longitudinal fasciculus and the tectobulbospinal system. It is difficult to distinguish the fibers of the medial longitudinal fasciculus (MLF) and the tectobulbospinal system (TBS) as they are so intimately intertwined. The central gray matter is seen to surround the central canal of the medulla with fibers of the hypoglossal and the dorsal motor vagal nuclei.

The level of the sensory decussation, so named due to the majority of the ascending sensory fibers decussating here, has the fibers of the dorsal column nuclei (cuneate and gracile) that originate just rostral to the motor decussation. It is at this point that the fiber conversion of the dorsal column to the gracile and the cuneate nuclei is evident. These paths are responsible for the impulses of the tactile and vibratory sensations of the body. Axons from the cuneate and gracile will continue as projections and become the internal arcuate fibers that will cross the midline as the sensory decussation and then continue as the medial lemniscal path on the contralateral side of the body. The topography of the path is arranged as follows, the lower extremity information is relayed within the gracile axon in the ventral aspect of the medial lemniscal path while the upper extremities information will be conveyed within the dorsal aspect medial lemniscal path via the cuneate fibers. Additional inputs are through the accessory cuneate nucleus that receives inputs via the cervical spinal nerves. These fibers will project to the cerebellum as cuneocerebellar fibers.

The lateral portion of the medulla houses the spinal trigeminal tract and the nucleus or pars articularis. The fibers from the ALS and the rubrospinal tract are seen to lie in the ventrolateral medulla. Inspection of the tissue will yield a bundle of fibers that lie adjacent to the ALS that are responsible for the spinal inputs that are then relayed on to the cerebellum. These tracts of fibers are called the lateral reticular nucleus. Other structures of the ventral medulla that require mention are the pyramid fibers, the hypoglossal nerve, and the inferior aspect of the inferior olivary complex. The hypoglossal nerve innervates the motor function of the ipsilateral aspect of the tongue. The solitary nucleus and the solitary tract receive sensory input from cranial nerves VII, XI, and X. The input is derived from the sensory dermatomes of thoracic and abdominal viscera and the carotid sinus.

Rostral to the obex the hypoglossal nerve and the dorsal vagal nuclei will make up the floor of the 4th ventricle. This is considered to be the level of the mid medulla. The restiform body now forms a large elevation on the dorsolateral aspect of the medulla. Within the elevation are the fibers of the dorsal Spinocerebellar, cuneocerebellar, olivocerebellar, reticulocerebellar fibers that will join as a conglomerate of fibers that together for the juxtarestiform body that will become the inferior cerebellar peduncle. Adjacent to the hypoglossal nucleus is the prepositus nucleus. This is the origin of the projections into the otic ganglion as peripheral fibers of the glossopharyngeal nerve.

Fibers at the level of the pons—medullary level will demonstrate some change in arrangement. The fibers of the restiform body will project superiorly to penetrate the cerebellum with the fibers of the facial motor nucleus aligning them ventrally. Adjacent to the facial nucleus will be the trapezoid body and the superior olivary nucleus. This is the level where the inferior olive will no longer be visible. Additional movement shows the medial lemniscal pathway moving into a more Ventrolateral position.

The medial medullary reticular area is made up of the central nucleus of the medulla and the gigantocellular reticular nucleus. Laterally, the medullary reticular area consists of the lateral nucleus and thus will form the parvicellular nucleus with the ventrolateral reticular area. The function of the parvicellular nucleus is in the regulation of the respiratory rates and heart rate. The nuclei raphe pallidus and the nucleus raphe magnus will receive the input of the central gray mesencephelon and project on to the spinal cord. The raphespinal fibers of the raphe magnus will modulate the inhibition of the pain sensations from the dorsal horn of the spinal cord.

The vertebral arteries, specifically the anterior spinal artery and posterior inferior cerebellar artery along with the posterior spinal artery will provide the majority of the blood supply to the medulla. The posterior inferior cerebellar artery will supply the dorsolateral medulla. The structures that are supplied by this artery will be the ALS, spinal trigeminal tract and associated nucleus, vestibular nuclei, solitary tract and its associated nucleus, the choroid plexus and the nucleus ambiguus. If there is insuffiency seen in the penetrating anterior cerebral arteries there will be contralateral hemiparesis in those structures innervated by the pyramidal and the corticospinal pathways. This hemiparesis is seen to be contralateral. There will be loss of proprioception and associated loss of vibratory sensation. The loss of vibratory sensation is due to the damage to the medial lemniscal pathway. If there is deficiency of circulatory supply to the area served by the posterior inferior cerebellar artery there is a characteristic pathology that will present itself. This pathology is called Wallenberg's syndrome. The presenting symptoms are contralateral loss of pain and temperature sensory inputs from the face with associated nystagmus, and loss of taste on the ipsilateral tongue.

CHAPTER 17

PONS

The pons are structures that are easily identified on the ventral surface of the brain between the midbrain and the medulla. The functional role of the pons is to be a relay center between the cerebral cortex and the cerebellum. By Latin definition, the word "pons" means to bridge. The neurons of the pons will receive the descending inputs from the cortex and then pass them along to the cerebellar cortex. These neurons are scattered throughout the ventral aspect of the brain. The pons are seen to be composed of several subdivision of tissue, the middle cerebellar peduncle or the brachium pontis and the basilar pons. There are a variety of nuclei associated with the pons and the pontomedullary junction. The nuclei are both sensory and motor nuclei and represent the abducens, the vestibular, the cochlear, the salivatory, the trigeminal, and the facial nuclei. The pons is easily identified as it has an unusual configuration as compared to the surrounding tissue. The fibers of the pons are arranged in a stacked horizontal array. The origin of the fibers is seen in the pontine nuclei and they will project across the midline. Some of the fibers will terminate the in the middle cerebellar peduncle and then eventually on into the cerebellum. The horizontally arranged fibers are termed the corticofugal fibers. These fibers will terminate in the spinal cord via nuclei of the brainstem, such as the tegmentum or directly on the pontine nuclei directly. There are also a set of "bumps' that are apparent with the pons as they are extensions of the facial colliculi. The corticopontine fibers have origins in the frontal, temporal, parietal and occipital lobes as they send projections to the ipsilateral terminations of the pontine nuclei. These pontine nuclei will in turn project on to the pontocerebellar fibers that will become the middle cerebellar peduncle as they project across the midline to the contralateral cerebellar cortex. Upon inspection of the surface markings and anatomy of the pons, there are cranial nerves seen to exit the brain along he pons, specifically the cerebellopontine angle. Examination of the surface anatomy will reveal cranial nerves V-VIII exiting the ventral surface of the pons. The lateral terminations of the middle cerebellar peduncle will become the penetrated by the Trigeminal Nerve. Upon inspection of the structural composition of the pons one can identify CN IV (abducens) as it exits the pons at the most medial aspect. The unique position of this cranial nerve is due to the proximity to the pyramidal tracts and the inferior pontine sulcus. As you move more laterally, CN VII (facial) will be seen to emerge in conjunction with CN VIII (vestibulocochlear) at the cerebellopontine angle. This angle is of major landmark importance as it is the demarcation between the joining of the medulla, the pons and the cerebellum.

Rostral to the spinal trigeminal nucleus will be the main sensory nucleus of the trigeminal nerve. This is seen at the level of the trigeminal nerve exiting the middle cerebellar peduncle. Inputs are from the cutaneous face. There will be inputs from all three of the large myelinated axons from the trigeminal ganglion that will enter the pons and terminate in the second order neuron of the main sensory nucleus. The organization of this is as the homunculus of the motor cortex as it is inverted in its relationship with the ophthalmic representations projecting ventrally while the mandibular representation is found laterally and the maxillary located between each of them. The secondary trigeminal projections will project as two (2) paths to the thalamic nuclei. The fibers that originate in the ventral aspect (ventrotrigeminothalamic fibers) of the sensory nucleus will cross midline and merge with the medial lemniscus pathway on their way to the contralateral VPM nucleus. The pain sensitive paths will differentiate from the dorsal portion of the main sensory nucleus. Upon the splitting off, the fibers will become the dorsal trigeminothalamic tract and provide the inputs for the ipsilateral mouth and tongue are represented in the ipsilateral thalamic nuclei. From this point the fibers will project on to the VPM and then on to the parietal operculum. These fibers relay the information for the touch, pressure sensations of the face and the intraoral cavity. This is in contrast to the motor nucleus fibers. These fibers are seen to occupy a position that is medial to the main sensory trigeminal nucleus. These neurons are also cholinergic in nature and the projections will take a position alongside the mandibular division of the trigeminal nerve. They are a completely separate nerve bundle however form the ventral fibers. The dorsal division will provide motor innervation to the muscles of mastication, the masseter, the anterior digastric, the mylohyoid and the tensor tympani. The corticobulbar fibers that were mentioned previously in this chapter will also project bilaterally to the trigeminal motor nuclei from the motor cortex. There are also mesencephalic trigeminal nuclei relays that are known to provide proprioception information for the jaw reflex to be elicited by the muscle spindles of the masseter muscle. There is also auditory input to the motor trigeminal nucleus that will then project to the tensor tympani to contract and thus dampen loud sounds via the stiffening of the middle ear ossicles.

The pontine tegmentum is defined by the composition of it. It contains several motor nuclei and many other groups of functionally related neurons. The central aspect of the pontine tegmentum is found to be composed mainly of the reticular formation, the central tegmental tract, and fibers that ascend from the reticular formation to the intralaminar nuclei as well as fibers that descend from the red nucleus to the inferior olive. The nucleus solitarius sends projections that will ascend through the tegmental tracts that provide information regarding taste to the thalamic nuclei. The facial nerve sends projections from the facial nucleus on the dorsolateral aspect of the pons. The facial nerve is also a unique structure in its own right as it has individual bindles of neurons. The neurons are bundled in motor and sensory packages. The motor bundle is larger than the sensory bundle and it is also often separated from the remaining two (2) sensory bundles by position. The positional change gives rise to the name of the sensory branch as the "intermediate nerve", due to the position it occupies between CN VII and CN VIII. The facial nerve fibers will project dorsomedially as they emerge from the facial nucleus and loop around the abducens nerve. CN VIII (vestibulocochlear) nerve is subdivided into motor and special sense. The superior cerebellar peduncle is the major efferent pathway of the cerebellum. Fibers from this origination will project rostrally into the midbrain. The fibers will decussate upon entering the brain.

In this arrangement, the medial lemniscus pathway will alter its position to a horizontal orientation in the tegmentum with the arm and the trunk in the medial aspect and the lower trunk and the lower extremities laterally. The spinothalamic path will ascend through the pons near the tip of the lateral portion of the medial lemniscus. This is important as brain stem bleeds or trauma will impose global deficit on the patient. Auditory fibers will enter the brainstem via the pontocerebellar angle and take a position more laterally with projection to a termination position that is in the dorsal and the ventral cochlear nuclei. The vestibular nerve fibers will follow those of the auditory fibers. The termination points of the vestibular nerves will differ and termination of these vestibular fibers will be in the four (4) vestibular nuclei. These nuclei occupy a position that is at the point of the fourth ventricle. These nuclei will fall to a position that is medial to the inferior cerebellar peduncle and yet dorsal to the spinal trigeminal nucleus and the nucleus solitarius. The vestibulocochlear nerve has a secondary set of neurons that will run in a slightly different path. Immediately ventral to the pontine tegmentum, the fibers will project into a transverse position and continue on into the trapezoid body. The trapezoid body is composed of decussating auditory fibers. These fibers will project on to the nuclei of the superior olivary complex. Not all of the fibers will follow this course as some of the fibers will project directly through the pons as the lateral lemniscus and the efferent projections from the superior olivary complex will merge into the lateral lemniscus and terminate in the inferior colliculus. There are projections from the juxtarestiform body that run along the dorsolateral regions of the fourth ventricle. The juxtarestiform body is a small collection of neurons that project on the fourth ventricle. There will be additional projections that will run the path to the spinal cord as the medial longitudinal fasciculus and extend to the pretectal area of the rostral brain. These fibers are along the midline and will project with motor nuclei of the extraocular muscles of the eye.

The organization of the medulla and the pons is not a haphazard array devoid of nuclei, but rather it is a highly organized aggregate of neurons. Centrally, the tegmentum is composed of the reticular formation composed of several nuclei. There is also the central tegmental tract that is found in the central aspect of the pontine tegmentum. This central tegmental tract is further composed of a variety of functional pathways. There are fibers from the reticular formation that will project to the intralaminar nuclei of the thalamus. Anatomists have revealed pathways that have origins in the rostral nucleus solitarius and project to the thalamus as they ascend the thalamic nuclei. These fibers are responsible for the conveyance of taste information. There are also descending fibers seen to project from the origins in the red nucleus to the inferior olive.

The nucleus of the abducens nerve is found anatomically along the midline of the brain inferior to the fourth ventricle. This nuclei is composed of two sets of neurons, a cholinergic collection of neurons and a collection of internuclear neurons. The nucleus is encased completely within the facial nerve as discussed previously in this chapter. The manner that the facial nerve encases the nucleus, produces the facial colliculus within the fourth ventricle. The internuclear neurons will emerge from the medial aspect of the nucleus and then project beyond midline and into the medial longitudinal fasciculus. The termination points are very specific for function in regards to the medial rectus muscle via the occulomotor complex. This is in direct opposition of the cholinergic neurons as they project directly to the lateral rectus muscle. The result of the activity of these two sets of neurons will be the production of a horizontal gaze.

The facial nucleus has several subdivisions associated with it as it rests in the caudal pons at the same level as the abducens nucleus within the ventrolateral reticular formation. Muscle innervation from the facial nucleus will include the platysma, the digastrics, the stapedius, buccinators and the other muscles of facial expressions. These are cholinergic neurons by convention. The relationship between the facial nucleus and the abducens nucleus is a very intimate one indeed, as the facial nucleus will encircle the abducens nucleus. Once this is achieved, the fibers will project to the cerebellopontine angle as described above. The facial nucleus also receives projections from the trigeminal nucleus. These projections are of major importance as they are responsible for the corneal reflex activity. This is due to the ophthalmic division of the trigeminal nerve. If the cornea is touched, the imputs are transmitted to the main sensory nucleus and the pars caudalis. There are other projections to the obicularis occuli that will regulate the blink reflex. The facial nuclei will also receive the projections from the facial motor component of the cerebral motor cortex and the premotor cortex. These are the corticobulbar fibers and in conjunction with portions of the reticular formation will provide multisynaptic inputs to the facial nucleus. The inputs that are sent are bilaterally sent if the motor cortex is regulating the upper face but only unilaterally sent if the imputs are for the contralateral lower face.

The salivatory nucleus is another cholinergic nucleus that is seen at the level of the pontomedullary junction. This nucleus has preganglionic fibers that are responsible for the regulation of saliva production. In the rostral medulla is the inferior salivatory nucleus deep within the lateral reticular formation. The end target of the preganglionic fibers will be the otic ganglion. Once in the otic ganglion, the final projection will be to the parotid gland where it will produce saliva. The afferent aspect of the salivatory reflex is acted upon by the rostral solitarius projections to the inferior salivatory nucleus. Before they complete the projection into the otic ganglion, the fibers will pass through the glossopharyngeal nerve and the lesser petrosal nerve. This is not the sole manner that the nervous system controls the production of saliva. The loose collection of cholinergic neurons located in the caudal pons will collectively originate as the superior salivatory nucleus. The fibers will project to the intermediate nerve to bifurcate at the geniculate ganglion of the facial nerve into the preganglionic fibers to the geniculate ganglion then to the chorda tympani to synapse on the postganglionic neurons of the Submandibular ganglion and then on to the submandibular and sublingual glands to produce saliva. The other branch of this bifurcation will go on to the greater Petrosal nerve to terminate in the pterygopalatine ganglion and then on to the lacrimal gland, the mucous lining of the nose and the mouth. The superior salivatory nucleus will have projections from the secondary trigeminal reflex to initiate the reflex release of tears with cornea irritation. The hypothalamus is the main regulator of the superior and the inferior salivatory nucleus by sending the descending fibers with the ANS being the system that is represented in this path.

CHAPTER 18

CEREBELLUM

The cerebellum is always associated with issues of motor disturbances. Experimental evidence has clearly demonstrated that it is involved in much more than just movement and movement disorders. Even with a relatively small percentage of the total mass of the human nervous system (~10%), the cerebellum is involved in many aspects of human activity. The cerebellum is however, the main resident of the posterior fossa. Protection for the cerebellum is also unique in that there is a tough fibrous protective layer extending over the dorsal aspect of it called the tentorium. The long understood and well defined role in the negative feedback aspect of movement is one aspect of the functional responsibility of the cerebellum. However, the cerebellum is also involved in the acceptance of multiple efferents from the periphery and the other input channels of the nervous system. The cerebellum is also involved in the integration of higher cognitive functioning as well as motor planning. Strangely as it may seem experimental resection in our lab demonstrated only limited paralysis and not long term. This is at odds with the expectations of the tissue mass given its initial role in motor coordination.

The cerebellum, as in the cerebral cortex demonstrates a layer array. Histologic inspection shows that there are anatomic divisions in the cerebellum as in the cerebrum as well. In the cerebellum, the fissures are the primary fissure, the posterior superior fissure, the prepyramidal fissure, the posterolateral fissure and the horizontal fissure. These (5) five fissures will divide the cerebellum into the lobes as the flocculonodular lobe, the anterior lobe and the posterior lobe. The cerebellum is divided into the vermis, a thin midline structure and flanked on either side by the hemispheres. The anterior lobe is composed of the lobules I-V. The posterior lobe is composed of lobules VI-IX. Anatomically, the folcculonodular lobe is composed of the nodus and the floccus collectively as lobe X. The cerebellum varies from the cerebrum in the anatomic term for the small gyri is "folia" rather than the gyri as noted in the cerebrum. The individual lobes are as noted above of lobules and in turn each lobule is composed of singular folium. Bundles of folium compose a folia. From a cellular perspective, the layers are composed of the Molecular layer, the Granular layer, and the Purkinje layer. The cerebellar cortex is a very highly convoluted structure. Inspection of the structures yields folia that are able to extend through and across the vermis. The adjacent anatomic structure is the brainstem. There are (3) three paired structures that are the tethering for the cerebellum and the brainstem that are known as the cerebellar peduncles. The inferior cerebellar peduncle is further composed of the restiform body found on the dorsolateral medulla at the level of the obex and the juxtarestiform body that is found on the wall of the fourth ventricle. The importance of these inferior cerebellar peduncle fibers and the interconnections they produce can be elicited from the origin of the fibers of this structure in the spinal cord or the medulla. The juxtarestiform body is seen to produce re

The Cebellar nuclei are seen within the central white matter of the cerebellum. The fastigial nucleus is also known as the medial Cerebellar nucleus. Anatomically, it is found to lie ini the midline and located on each lateral border will be the globose nucleus also known as the poster ior interposed nucleus and the emboli form nucleus also known as the anterior interposed nucleus. Functionally, the medial cerebellar nucleus is related to the cerebellar cortex while the anterior and posterior interposed nuclei are related to the intermediate zone of the cortex. The dentate nucleus is found to be lateral to the emboli form nucleus and is also known as the lateral cerebellar nucleus. Anatomically, the dent ate nucleus has a rosteromedial opening that is called the hilus. Compared to the other nuclei that are described in association with it the dentate nucleus is larger and this is attributed to the extreme size of the cortical zone it is known to overlie. From a functional point of view the dentate nucleus is associated with the lateral zone of the cortex.

The cerebellum just as the cerebrum is designed so that there are specific pathways of fibers designated to carry specific functional signaling. In the cerebellum, the cerebellar nuclei will be the origination of the bulk of the fibers designed to carry the effect signals. These axons are specific in characteristic function just as those in the cerebral cortex. These are defined as the cerebellar efferent projections. Biochemically, they demonstrate a grouping of neurotransmitter function, excitatory, and neurotransmitter utilized as being glutamate or aspartate. These neurotransmitters have been identified with excitatory functional characteristics and thus the function if these axonal pathways is upheld. The fastigial nuclei have histological origins within the fastigial nucleus, and they will send axonal projections Ina bilateral manner to the brainstem throu the juxtarestiform body. The superior cebellar peduncle is the exit point for the axonal projections frothe dentate nucleus, the emboli form nucleus and the globose nucleus. These fibers will demonstrate a characteristic crossing within the superior Cebellar peduncle that is different from other axonal projections. There will be collections of axons that will project on to the granular layer as the mossy fibers that have been given the name nucleocortical fibers. Histological studied have demonstrated them to provide excitatory inputs to the cerebellar cortex. If the fibers do not have origins within the cerebellar nuclei, they will demonstrate origins in the cerebellar cortex.

The cerebellar cortex has a layered arrangement as does the other aspects of the brain that has been discussed. The folium has been demonstrated to be composed of purkinje cell layer, a Granular layer and a molecular layer. The molecular layer is the outermost layer and it is composed of the least concentrated amount of cells as compared to the purkinje layer or the granular layers. The purkinje layer is also found to be adjacent to the white matter core. The purkinje cells are seen to exhibit a large cell body that may range from 40-70 um. The purkinje cell demonstrates extensive arborizations and these arborizations are special in that the terminal branches are responsible for the synaptic transmission of the cell. The terminal branches arise from the secondary and the teritary dendrites. The dendritic arbors will project into the molecular layer. These purkinje cells are the efferent projections of the cerebellum and they utilize GABA as the main neurotransmitter. These axonal projections will therefore present as a inhibitor of synaptic activity. The axons that arise from the purkinje cell is seen to originate from the basal aspect of the cell. These axons can project to the cerebellar corticonuclear fibers will arise from a variety of cortical areas. This is in contrast to the projections of the cerebellar corticovestibular nuclei as they arise vermis and the flocculonodular lobe.

The granular layer is composed of the small granule cell. The granule cell is small in comparison to the larger Purkinje cell as it is only 5-9 um. From a structural aspect, the cells of the granular layer are very distinct as they will project up into the molecular layer. The granular cells utilize glutamate and aspartate as the main neurotransmitters. The use of these amino acids as neurotransmitters clearly indicates an excitatory nature of the signals. This property is unique in itself as these are the only neurotransmitters that are found within the cerebellar cortex that are in fact excitatory. The granular cells demonstrate a cytoarchitecture that has the projecting axon bifurcate and make a 90 degree turn to project along the long axis of the folium, thus the naming parallel fibers. These axons also are seen to pass thought the densely populated purkinje layer while projecting synaptic connections along the way with the spiny branchlets of the purkinje cells. The cells of the granular layer are also seen to synapse with the cells of the molecular layer. The granular layer is also composed of cells called Golgi cells. There are some very distinct characteristics associated with these cells. First, the cell bodies are large, even larger than the granule cell, ranging to approximately 18-30um. Second, the chemical that they use as a neurotransmitter is GABA and not glutamate or aspartate. This is congruent with the characterization of function, as the Golgi are inhibitory in nature. These cells are also found in conjunction with the Purkinje cells.

Functionally, these cells are also seen to project into the molecular layer without regard to direction of projection. This layer is also the residence of the cerebellar glomerulus. the cerebellar glomerulus is a structure surrounded by glial cells, composed of a granule cell, Golgi cell axons and dendrites, and a mossy fiber.

The molecular layer is seen to have the least densely populated layer by volume, but has greatest population of projection. The cell types seen in this layer are the stellate and the basket cells. The neurotransmitter used in these cells are inhibitory in character as they use GABA as the chemical neurotransmitter. The stellate cells have subcatagorizations of superficial or outer stellate cells. These stellate cells are generally found at the most superficial aspect of the molecular layer. The cell bodies of the basket cell are seen to lie just superficial to the Purkinje cell layer. The cytoarchitecture of the basket cell is very similiar to that of the stellate cell in many ways, however the basket cell has a much broader receptive field than that of the stellate cell. The basket cell also has a much more braod scpoe of influence as compared to the stellate cell. Common features of the functional capacity of the stellate and basket cells is seen in the manner they receive inpulses from excitatory neurotransmitters of the parallel fibers. This holds true to the idea of the granule cell being the lone excitatory neuron within the cerebellar cortex. Another common aspect of the two cells is in the manner they distribute the influence in a sagittal plane and not as a projection into the upper layers of the cortex.

The afferent fibers that project into the cerebellar cortex are categorized into mossy fibers, multilayerd fibers (monoaminergic), and climbing fibers. The mossy fiber axons are seen to originate within the cerebellar nuceli as the nucleocortical fibers and these fibers have been identified as also having origins from other nuclei as well in the spinal cord, medulla and the pons. The mossy fibers obtain the cytoarcheticetural shape due to the rosettes of which there may be as many as 50 per mossy fiber. The neurotransmitter utilized by the mossy fiber is glutamate and thus it is excitatory in nature to the granule cell and the golgi cell. This use of the rosette in cellular configuration will allow for each rosette to then produce connections with up to 10-15 granule cells. The importance of this configuration is to expand the scope of influence of the mossy fiber tremendously. Additionally, the mossy fiber is able to project to other folia, again increasing the scope of influence of the mossy fiber. The rosette is the functional central component of the cerebellar glomerulus. The course that the projections will take on the path to the cortex is not always a direct one. There are many fibers that will produce collateral projections into the cerebellar nucleus.

The climbing fibers are known to have only a single origin. The climbing fiber utilizes the neurotransmitter aspartate and as such produces the excitatory effects on the Purkinje cell and the cerebellar nuclear cells. This sole origin of these climbing fibers is in the inferior olivary nucleus. These olivocerebellar fibers will produce collaterals that will then project on to the designated cerebellar nucleus. Termination of the climbing fibers is accomplished by actually climbing through the dendritic arbors of the Purkinje cells.

The monoaminergic multilayerd fibers are known to have origins in the locus ceruleus (noradrenergic), the raphe nuclei (seratoninergic), the hypothalamus (histaminergic) and a variety of other sites. The pathway that these fibers will take leads to the cerebellar cortex through the peduncles mainly. There will be other fibers projecting to the periventricular grey matter and then on to the cerebellum as the hypothalamocerebellar fibers. The unique aspect of these fibers is in the nervous system is in their ability to exert some influence on almost every cell type within the cerebellar cortex. This ability is due to the very extensive axonal projections into the molecular layer and the granular layers. Functionally, the influence described is in the inhibition of the discharge rate of the Purkinje cell, specifically, the spontaneous firing of the Purkinje cell. They also inhibit the influence of the climbing fibers and the mossy fibers on the Purkinje cells in a direct inhibition and also in a indirect manner via interneurons.

CHAPTER 19

LIMBIC SYSTEM

In the human nervous system, there are many things that we as neuroscientists and clinicians do not clearly understand the function and the manner of information flow. The limbic system is a major example of this type of tissue. The limbic system is unique for several reasons, first, that it receives inputs from many areas of the system as a whole and second, the vast array of behaviors that is demonstrates influence over. In order to provide this influence, the limbic system is composed of structural components that are adjacent to the limbus of the cerebral hemisphere and thus the name the limbic system. In laymens terms, the limbic system has become synonymous with emotion based function of the brain. This description of the function is true in many manners as the interconnections of the limbic system are known to influence emotional response to stimuli. The brain has been categorized by neuroscientists as either stimulating aversion centers or stimulating gratification centers. The limbic system is composed of minute yet well proliferated gratification and aversion centers. The cytoarchitecture demonstrates variability from tissue mass to tissue mass. Experimental evidence has shown the hippocampus and the amygdala to contain a predominance of aversion center tissue.

This is in direct contrast to the nucleus accumbens that has demonstrated a predominantly gratification structure.

Structurally, the limbic lobe is composed of the subcallosal region, the paraterminal gyri, the parolfactory gyri, the cingulate gyrus, the uncus, the parahippocampal gyrus, the hippocampal formation and the isthmus of the of the cingulate gyrus. These structures are aside from those that compose that limbic system, such as, the septal nuclei, the nucleus accumbens, hypothalamic mammilary nuclei, the amygdaloid complex, the substantia innominata, the dorsal thalamus, the habenular nuclei, the ventral tegmentum, the periaqueductal grey matter, the fornix, the stria terminalis, the ventral amygdalofugal paths, the mammilothalamic tract and the prefrontal cortex. Given the structures involved in the cytoarchitectural composition of the limbic system, it is easy to understand the sphere of influence that the limbic system can have.

The hippocampal formation is a large component of the limbic system and it is composed of Ammon's horn (hippocampus proper), subiculum laterally is found to be intertwined with the cortex of the parahippocampal gyrus and the dentate gyrus medially is seen to be interconnected with the fimbria of the hippocampus. In this configuration, the subiculum is actually a tissue of transition from the archicortex and the paleocortex. The archicortex is composed of the three layered hippocampus and the paleocortex is composed of the five layered parahippocampus. Histologically, the transition tissue is further subdivided into the prosubiculum, the subiculum, the presubiculum and the parasubiculum. These defining borders are somewhat ambiguous but are essential for the transfer or flow of inputs to the hippocampal formation and thus imperative structures. Damage to one of these structures can cause global implications.

The composition of the limbic system is complex and subdivisions are based on the embryologic development that is seen with this developmental sequence. The remnants of the hippocampus are provided by the migration of the limbic lobe into the final position in the temporal lobe. The is from the dorsal and ventral migration of the tissue mass that will produce the medial and the lateral longitudinal stria and the indusium griseum.

The Indusium griseum is the grey matter that is associated with both the medial and the lateral longitudinal stria. The external layer of the dentate gyrus and the hippocampus are both composed of three layer of cells and this external layer is the molecular layer with the middle layer being the granule cell layer in the dentate gyrus but the hippocampus it is called the pyramidal layer and then the inner is called the polymorphic layer.

Within the hippocampus, the inner layer, the alveus, is seen to lie adjacent to the wall of the lateral ventricle and it is unusual in that is is composed of myelinated fibers that have origins in the cell bodies of the subiculum and the hippocampus. The hippocampus is further divided into the C1, C2, C3 and C4 areas. In this instance the C is the designate for the embryologic origins of the tissue, the cornu ammonis from Ammon's horn. The C1 area is defined at the transition between the subiculum and the hippocampus and the C2 area is defined at the hippocampus proper as is C3 and the C4 designate is found to lie at the transition of the hippocampus and the dentate gyrus. These designations are important as the inputs to the hippocampus are through the perforant pathway. The axonal projections of the perforant pathway will terminate within the dentate gyrus, specifically the molecular cell layer. The termination is important as some of the cells will produce secondary terminations. The eventual terminal target is going to be the subiculum, along with projections from the amygdaloid complex. Some of the molecular cells will send continued projections on to the granular cells. The origins of the projections have been identified within the entorhinal complex. The terminal projections of the granular cells as noted above will project on to the molecular layer and on to the C1 region and subiculum via interneurons from C3 region. The fornix histologically is a cholinergic structure, the septohippocampal fibers are also destined for efferent projections to the hippocampus and the entorhinal complex. these are reciprocal circuits. The subiculum is a very important structure in as much as it is the main site for efferent projection. Axons will project from the subiculum and merge with axons from the pyramidal cells. These cells utilize glutamate as the neurotransmitter. The axons from both the subiculum and those from the pyramidal cell will continue on eventually becoming the fornix as the postcommissural fornix to final termination in the medial mammillary nucleus and hypothalamus. There are additional axonal projections that will continue on to the anterior nucleus of the dorsal thalamus. In the path that they take the axons will traverse the hippocampal decussation ventral to the splenum of the corpus callosum. Anatomically, the division of the pre and post commissural portions will be seen at the level of the anterior commissure. The fibers forming the precommisssural fornix have been shown to have origination in the hippocampus. The efferent projections are seen anatomically to project on into the septal nuclei, the nucelus accumbens, the preoptic area, and the anterior nuclei of the hypothalamus.

The almond shaped tissue found within the temporal lobe deep to the uncus is called the amygdala. Anatomically, this set of tissue has a composition that is made from a number of different nuclei and therefore the tissue conglomerate is called the amygdaloid complex. In dissection, the complex is found to lie in the rostromedial temporal lobe and specifically, rostral to the anterior temporal horn of the lateral ventricle. The composition of the tissue is defined by two subcategories, the basolateral and the corticomedial tissue groups. The basolateral group is associated with the higher cortical structures while the corticomedial group is associated with the sense of olfaction. The basolateral group is the larger of the two groups, however the corticomedial group is inclusive of the central nucleus.

The basolateral group is known to receive inputs from the dorsal thalamus, prefrontal cortex, parahippocampal gyrus, cingulate gyrus, insular cortex, parabracial nuclei, solitary nucleus, periaqueductal grey matter and the hypothalamus. The axonal projections from the basolateral cell group will reside in the medial aspect of the substantia innominata and some of these fibers will have terminal projections within the innominata as well as passing on to the hypothalamus and the septal nuclei. The fibers of the substantia innominata will cholinergic inputs on to the cerebral cortices. These projections will be to the frontal, prefrontal, cingulate gyrus, the insular and the inferior temporal corticies. There is tremendous experimental evidence of visceral inputs from the basolateral cell groups via the projection paths of the dorsal motor vagal, the raphe nuclei including the globus pallidus, the magnus, the obscures, the locus ceruleus, the parabrachial nuclei, and the periaqueductal grey matter. There is also additional pathways of influence on the brainstem for the basolateral cell group via the stria medullaris thalami as these projections move from the septal nuclei on to the habenular nuclei and then on as the habenulointerpeduncular tract. Additional projections from the amygdaloid complex are to the ventral amygdalofugal fibers and the stria terminalis. The stria terminalis was mentioned previously as it has origins in the corticomedial group. Anatomically, this tissue lies within a small groove that is created between the body of the caudate nucleus as it is adjacent to the dorsal thalamus. What is important about this tissue mass is the composition of the cells within it called the bed nucleus of the stria terminalis. The importance of the tissue mass is in the distribution of the fibers. This distribution is to the preoptic nuclei, ventromedial nucleus, the lateral hypothalamic region and the anterior nucleus. There are additional projections on to the septal nuclei, the caudate nucleus rostrally, the putamen and the nucleus accumbens. The tissue of the ventral amygdalofugal pathway has been identified as having origins in the basolateral group and the corticomedial cell group.

The small cell aggregation located rostral to the anterior commissure but within the wall of the septum pellicudium of the hemisphere is known as the septal region or the septal nuclei. The septal nuclei are relatively unknown for human function as there is evidence of the lesions of the area to produce uncontrolled rage anger. But this is a clinical scenario that is the result of a large lesion to the area. Inputs to the septal nuclei are seen to project from the fornix of the hippocampus, the stria terminalis and the amygdalofugal fibers of the amygdala, the ventral tegmentum, the preoptic area, the anterior, lateral and paraventricular hypothalamic nuclei. The efferent projection from the septal nuclei are then on to the septohippocampal area, habenular nuclei, the stria medullaris thalami, the preoptic, the anterior, the ventromedial and the lateral thalamic nuclei. The many reciprocal circuits are evident as the structures present both afferent and efferent projection to and from the septal nuclei. Therefore, this tissue mass, although small has global implications when lesioned. Many researchers believe that the projection from the medial forebrain bundle is perhaps the most important component of all. This mass of fibers will project on through the lateral hypothalamus and then on to the hypothalamus and on to the septum. It is via this mass of projections that there is communication with the brainstem. This is imperative as the neurotransmitter has been demonstrated to be dopamine and the effect is for the regulation of pleasure—drive reduction. This mechanism is important in how we achieve emotional regulation and balance.

The nucleus accumbens septi is found to lie within the rostral and ventral forebrain. Specifically, where the head of the caudate nucleus and the putamen are adjoined it is easiest to visualize the nucleus accumbens. This mass of neuronal tissue has been demonstrated to have influence on motor patterns and motor behaviors. This influence is actually exerted via a secondary mechanism and not as a direct influence. The ventral amygdalofugal path is the main input to the nucleus accumbens along with the hippocampus and the bed nucleus of the stria terminalis, and the medial forebrain bundle. The neurotransmitter that is associated to this tissue mass is unusual in that there are a variety of neurotransmitters including endogenous opiates that are used as the neurotransmitters. The outputs for the nucleus accumbens will project on to the hypothalamus, the globus pallidus, and the peduncles.

The limbic system has a role in the long term potentiation and memory. The experimental evidence suggests the long term potentiation at the individual synapses is the mechanism of action for the conversion of short term memory into long term memory. The neurotransmitter is glutamate. Release of the neurotransmitter will cause the NMDA-type glutamate receptor of the hippocampal cells to increase the influx of calcium ions that will in turn increase the nitric oxide to diffuse back to the presynaptic cell. This will produce a increase in the release of glutamate on a permeant basis. This is how the theory of long term potentiation comes about, having a single cell stimulated with exponential results.

CHAPTER 20

SPINAL PATHWAYS

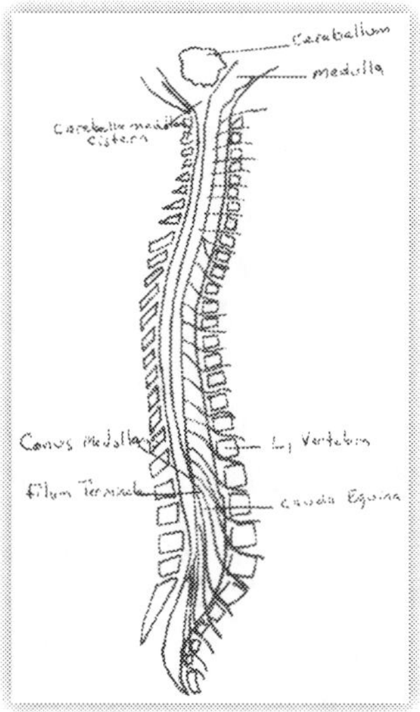

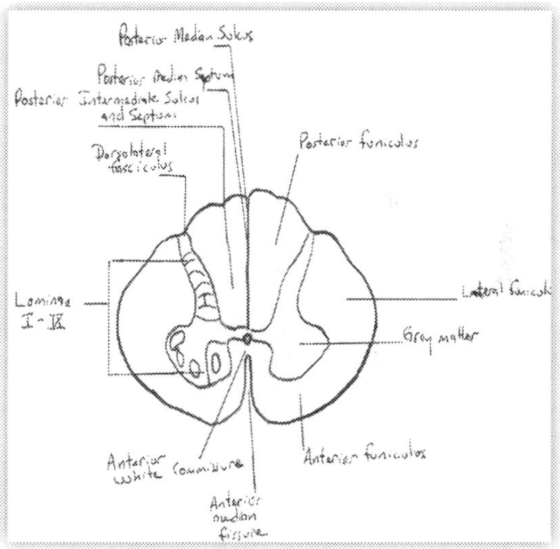

The organization of the human nervous system is grouped in a methodical manner. The spinal cord is grouped into fiber tracts that are either ascending or descending tracts. These tracts are also grouped according to positional or topographical arrangements. The organization of the system also allows for the manner anatomists and neuroscientists name the paths, utilizing origin, termination ascending or descending properties to produce descriptive names of the pathways. This allows for distinct sets of tissue to be compartmentalized into a particular aspect or position within the cord. If the fibers have the same origin—path—and terminal point they are known as tracts or as fasciculi. In general terms we can say the following "DAS-VEM" Dorsal—Afferent-Sensory & Ventral—Efferent-Motor. The spinal cord is subdivided into three funiculi and this arrangement contains the ascending and descending tracts to be held within one or more of these three funiculi. This topographic arrangement of fibers leads to the following collections; shorter tracts are located more centrally in the grey matter while the longer tracts are found to lie more peripherally in the white matter of the spinal cord. By the axiom "DAS-VEM" the Dorsal—Afferent-Sensory portion indicates that the ascending fibers are located in the dorsal aspect and would therefore transmit sensory afferent impulses. Let us look to see if this is correct in our assumption.

ASCENDING PATHWAYS

ANTERIOR SPINOTHALAMIC PATHWAY

Anatomically, we see that the ascending tracts transmit impulses associated with the stretch receptors, the tactile receptors and the projections are to either the interneuron nuclei or directly to the cerebellum. This supports the statement we made. Histologic examination reveals that the anterior spinothalamic tract has origins within the spine at the spinal grey matter, specifically in the lamina I, IV and V contralaterally. As the path ascends, they are seen to rise and then cross to the terminal points within the thalamus. The fibers of the anterior spinothalamic tract are found within the anterior and the anterolateral funiculi. Within the composite of the anterolateral funiculi, the fibers that have origins in the sacral and the lumbar areas are found to be more laterally placed while those that have origins within the cervical and the thoracic areas are more medially located with the uncrossed fibers holding the most medial placement. The fibers of the spinothalamic path will ascend and cross within the anterior white commissure at multiple levels thus producing a variant in the pathologic presentation with single versus multiple level injury. This configuration of fibers will differentiate some as the anterior spinothalamic path and these fibers will ascend within the anterior funiculi and the anterolateral funiculi as mentioned above. It is important to understand this arrangement as at the level of the midbrain, the anterior spinothalamic path will differentiate into two distinct subdivisions. The section that is located most lateral will be found terminating in the ventral posterolateral pars caudalis (VPL_c) thalamic nuclei. This is in contrast to the section that is found medially as it is found to terminate within the periaqueductal grey matter and then on to the intralaminar thalamic nuclei. The function of the anterior spinothalamic nuclei is to produce and elicit interpretation of the "light touch" tactile input.

LATERAL SPINOTHALAMIC PATHWAY

The lateral spinothalamic path differs from the anterior not only in the course of the fibers but the sensory information conveyed as well differentiates this from the anterior path. This path is assigned the task of conveying the sense of pain and thermal information. The fibers of this path are also seen to send projections on the reticular formation while the main fibers are destined for the VPL_c fibers of the thalamus. The cells of this path that have been demonstrated to have origins in the Lamina I, IV and V will have the same course as those mentioned above for the spinothalamic fibers. They will cross in the anterior commissure; they will ascend in the contralateral lateral funiculus but now as the lateral spinothalamic tract. The path is seen to occupy a position that is medial to the spinocerebellar tract in cross section. The manner that the fibers are seen to cross the spinal cord is different than that of the anterior spinothalamic path as well. The fibers of the lateral spinothalamic path will cross to the contralateral side at or within one spinal level. However, this group of fibers is also topographically arranged just as the anterior spinothalamic path.

SPINOTECTAL PATHWAY

The origins of the spinotectal fibers are seen within the laminae I and V within the posterior horn of the spinal cord. From a structural point of view, the fibers are seen to ascend within the same anterolateral aspect of the spinal cord as was discussed in the spinothalamic pathway. Anatomically, the differentiation of the pathways becomes evident within the midbrain as the fibers of the spinotectal pathway pass along to the periaqueductal grey matter as well as the superior colliculus. From a functional point of view, the pathway has implications in the visual system via the inputs to the colliculus and implications in the perceptive aspect of pain transmission.

ANTERIOR SPINOCEREBELLAR PATH

The anterior spinocerebellar pathway has been demonstrated to have origins within the lumbar spine as a collection of non-distinct cells within the lamina V, VI and VII. Inspection of the pathway will show a non-crossed arrangement as the fibers ascend the spinal cord. Functionally, the fibers of this pathway are concerned with the motor control and postural inputs from the lower extremity as a whole. Supportive evidence of the naming of the pathway as the spinocerebellar pathway is clear. Anatomically, the fibers occupy a position that is on the periphery of the dorsal aspect of the cord. Given the origination of the cells that make up this pathway, the functional capacity of the pathway should not surprise the reader to be of lower extremity origins into the nervous system. The representation of the inputs is seen to be from the monosynaptic firing of the Ib afferents (DAS—Dorsal—Afferent-Sensory) form the Golgi tendon Organ found within the muscle spindles of the joints of the lower extremity. The experimental evidence supports the fact that the muscles whose inputs are transmitted are synergistic muscles of the joint whose inputs are transmitted. The anatomic composition of the pathway as it projects on to the cerebellum is made up of the first neuron (1) within the spinal ganglia and the second neuron (2) intersparsed cells within the lumbar, sacral and coccygeal aspects of the anterior and posterior horns. The second neuron fibers (2) have been demonstrated histologically to cross in the cord to occupy a position that is superficial to the lateral spinothalamic tract until the fibers project to the upper pons. It is at the upper pons that the path will enter the cerebellum to the superior cerebellar peduncle and then on to the contralateral anterior cerebellar vermis in lobules I, II, III and IV.

POSTERIOR SPINOCEREBELLAR PATHWAY

The fibers of the posterior spinocerebellar pathway will ascend the cord in a position within the posteriolateral aspect of the cord. The origins of this pathway are seen in the Dorsal nucleus of Clarke The cells of this nucleus are the origins of the large fibers that will project in the posterolateral aspect of the lateral funiculus. There is a unique feature that is seen in this pathway from a structural stand point, that being the association of the fibers into the inferior cerebellar peduncle as they project to the termination within the caudal aspect of the cerebellum vermis ipsilaterally. Upon entering the cerebellum, the fibers will bifurcate and send projections that remain ipsilateral but show anterior and posterior components. The anterior component will terminate within the lobules I, II, III and IV while those demonstrated to occupy the posterior position will terminate in the pyramis and the paramedian lobule. The anatomic distinctions between the anterior and the posterior spinocerebellar pathways is important anatomically, but also important functionally. The fibers of the posterior spinocerebellar pathway will carry impulses from the muscle spindles, Golgi tendon organs as well as the receptors for touch and pressure. The difference between the pathways is seen in the neurons that are monosynaptically activated are done so via the Ia, Ib and II afferent fibers. The inputs are via the dermis, and the postural activity and as such the regulation from the pathway is involved in the fine coordinated motor movements, posture, and pressure discrimination. There is an important difference in the sensory inputs of the skin here as well as those from the anterior spinocerebellar pathway in that the posterior fibers have experimentally been shown to work in the manner we adapt to pressure, more specifically the slow manner we adapt to those pressure sensations.

CUNEOCEREBELLAR PATHWAY

The cuneocerebellar pathway is found to lie within the fasciculus cuneatus. The fibers of this pathway are uncrossed as they ascend on to the accessory cuneate nucleus of the medulla and enter the cerebellum through the inferior cerebellar peduncle to continue on to the final termination within the lobule V of the cerebellar cortex. The functional aspect of the cuneocerebellar pathway is for the input of movement and postural sensory data. The cuneocerebellar pathway is also responsible for the pressure discrimination as described in the posterior spinocerebellar pathway, by slow adaptation to the pressure stimuli.

SPINORETICULAR PATHWAY

The spinoreticular pathway is seen to have origins in the posterior horn of the spinal cord. These ascending fibers will travel within the anterolateral portion of the spinal cord to the final termination within the nucleus reticularis gigantocellularis of the medulla's reticular formation. There are a small number of fibers that have been demonstrated to continue on to the midbrain reticular formation. And another small group of fibers will pass on to the pontine reticular formation. The fibers of this pathway have been demonstrated to be uncrossed. From a functional point of view, the spinoreticular pathway is involved in the modulation of behavior and motor-sensory activities.

SPINO-OLIVARY PATHWAY

The spino-olivary pathway has two distinct subdivisions, the anterior and the posterior paths. These fibers are seen to travel along the posterior white column with synaptic connections in the nucleus cuneatus and the nucleus gracilis with final projections on to the accessory olivary nucleus. Excitation of this pathway is via the cutaneous Ib receptor. The anterior spino-olivary fibers are seen to ascend contralaterally within the anterior funiculus with final termination in the dorsal and the medial accessory olivary nuclei which then will in turn send projections on to the olivocerebellar fibers that are seen as crossed fibers pushing on to the anterior lobe of the cerebellum.

POSTERIOR WHITE COLUMNS

Anatomically, there are fibers with origins in the cells of the spinal ganglia that bifurcate and form long ascending pathways and short descending pathways that collectively are called the Posterior White Columns. These fibers will convey the sense of touch and pressure as well as kinesthesia. This is the pathway investigated when assessment is made of the patients two point discrimination capacity. This pathway also houses the group Ia muscle spindle afferents as well as the group Ib Golgi tendon organ afferents. Histologic examination will elicit a pattern of fiber arrangement that will have the fibers with origins from the cervical dorsal roots being found lateral to those with origins in the thoracic dorsal roots. This positioning of the fibers will elicit a layered configuration of the pathways. In this configuration, the layering is called laminar arrangements, and upon examination, the overlapping of fibers will have the longer sacral fibers occupying the most medioposterior position while the shorter cervical fibers are found to occupy the most lateral position and the intermediate position being found occupied by the lumbar and the thoracic fibers. The posterior funiculus is seen to be divided at the T6 level by the posterior septum at within the upper thoracic and the cervical areas of the spinal cord. The septum is seen to run longitudinally along the spinal cord as it divides the fasciculus gracilis on the medial aspect from the fasciculus cuneatus laterally. Both the fasciculus gracilis and the fasciculus cuneatus will ascend the spinal cord ipsilaterally. As the fibers ascend the cord they are seen to terminate within the nucleus gracilis and the nucleus cuneatus in a topographic arrangement. From this terminal point the nuclei will send second order neurons that will become the internal arcuate fibers. These fibers will cross and join to form the medial lemniscal pathway and continue on via the contralateral brain stem to their final terminal point within the ventral posterolateral nucleus and the pars caudalis of the thalamus (VPL_c). In order to better understand the structural aspect of the pathways, a better understanding of the first versus second order neurons is helpful. The spinal ganglion cells have a central process that is seen to penetrate the spinal cord and climb ipsilaterally within either the fasciculus cuneatus or the fasciculus gracilis. These neurons are called the first order neurons because the fibers will terminate within the cells of the nucleus gracilis or the nucleus cuneatus of the posterior column. The fibers that then will project from the nucleus and cross within the deep medulla and will make up the medial lemniscus then project on to the contralateral thalamus are the second order neurons.

DESCENDING COLUMNS

TECTOSPINAL PATHWAY

The cells of this pathway are identified as having origins within the internal superior colliculus. The fibers of this pathway are associated with reflex postural movements that are in conjunction with the inputs from the visual system and the auditory system. The fibers will then project along the periaqueductal grey matter to cross midline within the dorsal tegmental decussation to continue on in the median raphe just anterior to the medial longitudinal fasciculus. The fibers once they reach the spinal cord will occupy a position within the anterior funiculus adjacent to the anterior median fissure. The neurons of this pathway are only seen in the cervical portion of the spinal cord (C1-5) and are seen with terminal points at Lamina VI, VII, and VIII.

MEDIAL LONGITUDINAL FASCICULUS (MLF)

This is a unique pathway as the cellular origin is a variant of multiple origins of multiple nuclei from the brain stem. These cells will send projections that will conjoin into a bundle as the MLF. These variable origins are from the pontine reticular formation (the largest contributor of fibers), the medial and the inferior vestibular nuclei, superior colliculus and the interstitial nucleus of Cajal as these fibers project from the mesencephalic nucleus lateral to the Occulomotor complex and the MLF. The fibers of the interstitial nucleus of Cajal are known to project in an uncrossed manner all the way to the termination in lamina VII and VIII. This bundle of neurons is visible mainly within the cervical spinal levels but the pathway does project the length of the cord into the sacral segments. These fibers are in contrast with those of the medial vestibular nucleus as these fibers have been demonstrated to run ipsilaterally within the spinal cord as they send projections on to the laminae VII and VIII.

CORTICOSPINAL PATHWAY

This is one of the most complex pathways within the brain and the spinal cord. The main neurotransmitters of this pathway are the amino acids glutamate and aspartate. The complexity arises from the many different origins of cells for the pathway and also from the manner that they traverse the brain on the way to the terminal points. The origin of the pathway comes from the cells within the cerebral cortex. The origins of this path are seen in the premotor, motor area, postcentral gyrus and the lamina V cells. The organization within the areas shows a very close compacted linear array, such that it forms strips of origin cells. From a cytoarchitectural design, the largest of the cells of origin are those from the Betz cells (pyramidal cells) found within the precentral gyrus. Histological examination shows the fibers that project from these cells will form a portion of the corona radiate to project through the internal capsule and final project to the crus cerebri within the midbrain. These fibers will continue along to their termination along a path within the infratentorial brainstem adjacent to the 4th, 6th and the 12th cranial nerve. Histologically, the medullary pyramids are composed of the majority of these fibers as they project into the spinal cord as they decussate along this margin. These projecting fibers are unique in that they undergo incomplete decussation in order to produce three (3) separate pathways. The pathways that are produced are the uncrossed small anterior corticospinal path, the very large crossed lateral corticospinal pathway, and finally the uncrossed anterolateral corticospinal pathway. The lateral corticospinal pathway has some characteristics that allow the identification of the fibers as they sit within the spinal cord. These fibers will run the entirety of the spinal cord, sending out projections at each spinal gray level. Unique to the path, are the projection from the sacral and the lumber segments that will project around to the dorsolateral aspect of the spinal cord. There are fibers that will project in the intermediate zone as they continue into the Lamine IV, V, VI and VII. These are in contrast to the fibers of the anterior corticospinal pathway that is uncrossed in its course into the spinal cord to rest along the anterior median fissure as they project to termination in laminae VII. The decussation of these fibers will be at the upper cervical spinal levels within the anterior white commissure.

The uncrossed anterolateral pathway fibers are seen to terminate in the posterior horn and in the intermediate grey matter.

RUBROSPINAL PATHWAY

The origin of this pathway is identified as being from the magnocellular cells of red nucleus of the midbrain tegmentum. The red nucleus is seen to have efferent projections to it from the cerebellar peduncle in a crossed projection. Stimulation of the red nucleus elicits excitatory post synaptic activity in contralateral flexor alpha motor neurons and inhibitory post synaptic activity in the extensor alpha motor neurons. These pathway fibers will decussate within the ventral tegmentum decussation to project on to the cervical and lumbar aspects of the spinal cord. Those fibers that are projecting into the cervical aspects are seen to originate within the dorsomedial red nucleus while those that project in to the thoracic portion of the spinal cord have been demonstrated as having origins within the intermediate portion of the red nucleus and those projecting to the lumbosacral aspect of the spinal cord are seen to originate within the ventrolateral aspect of the red nucleus. The main function of the pathway is in the regulation of the flexor tone of the muscles.

VESTIBULOSPINAL PATHWAY

This grouping of fibers has a unusual configuration that is found within the floor of the fourth ventricle within the pons and the medulla. The pathway is seen to modulate the somatic spinal reflex activity for extensor muscle tone via the extensor alpha motor neuron. The cellular origins of this pathway are within the giant cells of the lateral vestibular nuclei. This pathway is seen to project ipsilaterally in the spinal cord within the anterior lateral funiculus as it passes along the entire length of the spinal cord. The somatotopic organization of the fibers demonstrates a dorsocaudal and rostroventral arrangement with the dorsocaudal fibers projecting to the lumbosacral spinal segments via the monosynaptic excitation of the gamma motor neurons and the rostroventral fibers projecting on to the cervical spinal segments. There are extensive interconnections with the Laminae VII and VIII via the interneurons.

SPINAL PATHWAYS

DESCENDING PATHWAYS

PATHWAY	FUNCTION	SIDE
ANT. CORTICOSPINAL	Skilled movements	Contralateral
MEDIAL LONGITUDINAL FASCICULUS		Same
MEDULLARY RETICULOSPINAL VENTROLATERAL	Automatic Respirations	Same
RUBROSPINAL	Flexor MM tone	Same
VESTIBULOSPINAL	Extensor MM tone	Same
LATERAL CORTICOSPINAL PYRAMIDAL	Skilled movements	Same

ASCENDING PATHWAYS

FASCICULUS GRACILIS	Joint position, fine touch vibration	Same
ANT. SPINOTHALAMIC	Light touch	Contralateral
FASCICULUS CUNEATUS	Joint position, fine touch Vibration	Same
SPINOTECTAL	Nocioceptive	Contralateral
ANT. SPINOCEREBELLAR	Whole limb position	Contralateral
LAT. SPINOTHALAMIC	Pain & temp	Contralateral
POST. SPINOCEREBELLAR	Stretch receptors	Same

COMBINATION PATHWAYS

DORSOLATERAL FASCICULUS OF LISSAUER		Ascending/Descending
FASCICULUS PROPRIUS	Short spinospinal paths	Ascending/Descending

CHAPTER 21

BRAIN TUMORS

Tumors of the human nervous system are classified by the current world Health Organization classification of tumors. This listing provides a comprehensive system for the universal discussion of tumors with regards to size, origin, type of growth etc. Intracranial tumors are tumors that have origins within the cranium, meningeal coverings, pituitary and or pineal gland, brain cortex, cranial nerves, blood vessels, metastatic origins and congenital origins. Many texts will include the parasitic cysts, granulomas and lymphomas as well. The most common clinical complaints of a patient are ranked as the following: a progressive change in neurologic status (68%), headache (54%), and finally progressive motor weakness (45%). Intracranial tumors are further subdivided into nine subclassifications:

1. Cranium-Cranial Nerve Tumors

Osteomas
Hemangiomas
Hyperostosis

Granulomas
Osteitis deformans
Xanthomatosis

2. Gliomas
3. Pineal Tumors—Pituitary Tumors
4. Cranial Nerve Tumors
5. Meningeal Tumors

Meningiomas
Gliomatosis
Metastatic Origin
Sarcomatosis

6. Congenital Tumors

Teratomas
Chordomas
Craniopharyngiomas
Cholesteatomas
Dermoids
Cysts

7. Metastatic Tumors
8. Granulomas
9. Blood Vessel Tumors

Angiomas
Hemangioblastomas

Intracranial tumors are also classified according to location in regards to the tentorum cerebelli. Therefore they are either supratentorial or infratentorial tumors. The symptoms and outcomes of these types of tumors are varied and will be reviewed here. The incidence rate of the intracranial tumors is greater in men than in women. The rate of the tumor being metastatic is greater the later in life the individual is at the time of diagnosis. The concern of any type of tumor is alterations in the pressure within the closed cranium. Since the brain is encased within the hard cranium, any alteration in the pressure that is seen within the cavity can produce significant pathology and possibly become incompatible with life. The symptoms of intracranial tumor are seen to vary according to location, size infiltration of surrounding tissue and increases in intracranial pressure. Incidence rates of brain tumors in children run approximately 4:100,000. The most common types of tumors in children are cerebellar gliomas, pineal tumors, optic nerve tumors, brain stem tumors, teratomas, craniopharyngiomas and meduloblastomas (primitive neurectodermal tumors).

CHAPTER 22

MUSIC ASSOCIATION AND LEARNING

Complex sounds are mixtures of pure tones that are either harmonically related, thus having pitch or randomly arranged, as noise. Sound is a mechanical disturbance that is propagated through an elastic medium. This medium is usually air but it is possible to be liquids, viscous materials or even solids. In humans, the cochlea is the portion of the system that changes sound waves into audible neurologic signals. It functions by the ability to analyze the sounds by separating the complex waveforms into individual frequencies. Any variation in pressure as a function of time is called a sound wave. This wave is representative of the characteristics of the population of molecules as a whole rather than as a single molecule. The relationship between the wavelength (λ), conduction velocity (c), and frequency (f) is expressed as cycles / second = hertz (Hz). In this mathematical model, the frequency of a wave (f) is expressed as cycles per second while the period (T), is equal to the time interval between the peaks of a wave. This is expressed in the following equation ($\lambda = c / f$, with f being $= 1/T$). In the interpretation of the sound, the brain will obtain directional origin from the computational differences in the shape, timing and intensity of the waveforms that reach the ear.

This interaural time difference (ITD) is calculated by the formula (D_1-D_2) V = ITD. Interaural time and intensity differences are related to the angle between the directions in which the sound source is in relation to the direction of the head, specifically, the pinna of the ear. The interaural time differences are more important for the localization of the low frequency sound waves whilst the intensity differences are most important in high frequency sounds.

MECHANISM OF HEARING

The sound capturing device of the human body is the ear. The ear is anatomically divided into three aspects. The outer ear or the external ear, the middle ear, and the inner ear are the anatomic divisions of the ear. Sound will be captured by the outer ear to travel along the external auditory meatus for transposition upon the tympanic membrane. As the sound waves contact the tympanic membrane, there is a disturbance generated from the sound wave that will create oscillation of the tympanic membrane. This oscillation will in turn generate vibration in the ossicles (bones) that will conduct the mechanical energy of the oscillation to the oval window of the cochlea. As the cochlea receives this oscillation, it will transfer the mechanical energy of the sound wave to the fluid filled compartment. This distribution of mechanical energy will continue to be transferred to the basilar membrane. This membrane will translate the mechanical energy into electrochemical energy through the activation of the Organ of Corti. These hair cells will be stimulated through the mechanical waves described previously and stimulate the attachment points to initiate the electrochemical release from the receptors.

The outer ear is consistent of the actual outer ear or the pinna and the external auditory meatus. The function of the external ear, the pinna is to collect and direct sound waves into the external auditory meatus. High frequency sound waves, those > 5 Hz or more, are affected by the pinna. The pinna is important in localization of sounds in the vertical plane more than any other direction. The middle ear is made up of the tympanic membrane or the ear drum and the 3 bony ossicles, the malleus, the incus and the stapes.

The function of the middle ear is impedance matching. Impedance matching is a very complex process that is designed to reduce the loss of energy as the sound waves are conducted through the system. The actual mechanism of the impedance matching is the mechanical advantage from the reduction of the surface area from the tympanic membrane to the ossicles. The point of consolidation is the footplate of the stapes. This reduction of surface area will elicit a pressure amplification of 20:1 or 30:1. Experimental evidence has demonstrated a loss of the transfer of energy in this aspect of the ear to be near 99%. How this amplification takes place is an energy expenditure of adenosine triphosphate as the tiny muscles of the middle ear, the tensor tympani and the stapedius muscle contract and relax. Innervation of the tensor tympani is from the motor division of the trigeminal nucleus and the innervation of the stapedius muscle is from the motor nucleus of the facial nerve. In the actions of these muscles, the stiffness of the bony chain of the ossicles will be directly influenced. As the muscles contract, making the chain of bone more stiff, there is a dampening effect on the transmission of the sound waves as mechanical energy through these bones. If the muscles are to contract maximally, there is a possible reduction of the sound by 15-20 decibels. Anatomically, the bony ossicles are configured with the arm of the malleus is attached to the tympanic membrane and footplate of the stapes found to be attached to the oval window at the opposite end. The tympanic cavity is an air filled cavity located within the middle ear, specifically, the temporal bone. It is found to lie within between the tympanic membrane and the inner ear.

The inner ear is divided into three inter connected parts, the semicircular canals, the vestibule and the cochlea. The cochlea as discussed previously is designed to be the frequency filter that will separate and analyze the sound frequency. The cochlea is a membranous tissue encased within an osseous portion. It consists of three spiraling chambers. The base of the cochlea (closest to the middle ear) being connected to the saccule of the membranous labyrinth by the ductus reunieuns and connected to the apex at the opposite end. Internally, the cochlea is fluid filled and divided by the basilar membrane along its longitudinal axis. This basilar membrane will create three compartments within the cochlea. These compartments are the scala vestibule, the scala tympani and the scala media. The central chamber of the cochlea is the cochlear duct. The cochlear duct or the scala media is bound inferiorly by the basilar membrane and superiorly by the vestibular membrane or Reissner's membrane and the stria vascicularis externally. More superiorly is the scala vestibule that communicates with the vestibule, the portion of the inner ear that is found between the oval window and the cochlea. Inferiorly, lies the scala tympani. The scala tympani is seen to terminate at the oval window and is the demarcation between the cochlea and the middle ear cavity. The screw like shaped portion of the inner core of the cochlea is the modiolus. The scala vestibule and the scala tympani are filled with perilymph while the cochlear duct (scala media) is filled with endolymph. The production of the endolymph is from the stria vascularis.

As the pressure wave travels along the length of the cochlea, it will create a pressure differential across the basilar membrane. This differential is visualized between the scala vestibule and the scala tympani. By generating this pressure differential, there will be generation of a mechanical wave that will produce a vibrational wave moving as a traveling wave. The traveling wave will contact the basilar membrane and as this is linked through anatomic attachment to the spiral ligament, generate the transmission of the mechanical energy to the ligament. The wave energy is then transferred at the point of the round window to the scala tympani.

The Organ of Corti consists of specialized epithelium that is set upon the basilar membrane. The Organ of Corti has two very specialized epithelial cells. These cells are specialized receptors. The first of these two cells are the inner and outer hair cells and the second specialized receptor being the tectorial membrane. These structures are found within the scala media and are attached to the basilar membrane. The basilar membrane is a very unique structure in the manner it produces a variable grade of stiffness. This basilar membrane is a relatively flaccid structure that increases in width and decreases in stiffness from its base to apex. These hair cells are connected to the tectorial membrane. Functionally, as the sound waves pass through the compartment, they create a mechanical disturbance that is translated in to the inner ear establishing a mechanical disturbance along the basilar membrane and the Organ of Corti. This mechanical disturbance is a wave of vibration. The result of this vibration is displacement will be a shearing force applied to the tectorial membrane and concurrently to the hair cells. The shear force applied to the hair cells will result in depolarization of the cell and eventual release of neurotransmitter. By the stimulation of the hair cell, there is the point of conversion of the mechanical energy into electrochemical energy. Until this shear force is applied to the hair cell, the system input has been all mechanical energy. It is important to distinguish that this is the point of the exchange of the mechanical energy to conversion into electrochemical energy. The conversion is through the hair cell being innervated by the peripheral branches of the axons of the bipolar neurons whose cell bodies are located in the spiral ganglion and the central axons that make up the auditory nerve. As the impulse is continued along this energy conversion, the impulse will continue as an action potential within Cranial Nerve 8, the vestibulocochlear nerve. If there are two sound waves that become passed along to the cochlea at the same time, each sound wave will create it's own maximal displacement at particular points of the basilar membrane. The basal portion of the membrane responds to the higher frequencies while the lower frequencies are known to create maximal displacement at the apical portions of the membrane.

The Inner hair cells are a single line of spiraling hairs that run from the apex to the base of the membrane. The outer hair cells will form three parallel lines that will run following the exact same course. The structure of the hair is such that the apical portion of the hair demonstrates a long projection called the hair bundle. This hair bundle consists of between 50 to 150 stereocilia. The inner hair cells are separated from the outer hair cells by the Tunnel of Corti.

The Tectorial membrane is a gelatinous membrane that is seen to extend over the sensory epithelium from the limbus of the osseous spiral lamina. The taller stereocilia are embedded within the Tectorial membrane. The central processes of the spiral ganglion cells will form the cochlear portion of the vestibulocochlear nerve. The efferent fibers to the cochlea either spiral along the inner part of the basilar membrane to synapse on the inner hair cells or they will travel along radially to the Tunnel of Corti to contact the outer hair cells. Therefore the response of the hair cells will be greatest at the point of the greatest displacement of the hair cell and the tectorial membrane.

A particulat set of fibers will be activated by a pure tone. When the tone changes frequency, the population of the nerve cells that is stimulated will change in accordance with the tone change. This alteration of the nerve cell stimulation is called the place principle of hearing. This principle states that the perceived pitch of a sound depends only on the particular population of neural elements that are activated. The actual mechanoelectrical transduction comes from the inner hair cells that convert the mechanically applied force from the hair bundle into the electrical signal through the displacement of the hair that is secondary to the sound wave and the creation of the pressure differences within the cochlea. Compositionally, the endolymph has an increased potassium concentration [K^+]. This is in direct opposition to the content of the perilymph that has increased concentration of [Na^+]. The displacement of the tectorial membrane will create a displacement of the hair bundles and therefore the stereocilia that is in contact with the tectorial membrane will have displacement as well from the attachment with the anchoring points that are connected to the nerve endings of the cochlear nuclei. When the hair bundles are displaced, they in turn will stimulate the attachment points and allow the opening of the potassium channels within the receptors stimulated by the stereocilia and by the increased permeability of the receptor to potassium result in cell depolarization. If there is damage to the stria vascularis, there will be resultant loss in the endolymph electric potential and following failure of the action potential to propagate. As the hair cell depolarizes, the voltage gated calcium channels at the bases of the cells will open and the release of the neurotransmitter will follow.

As discussed previously, differing regions of the cochlea will respond to different frequencies. The basilar membrane exhibits cross striations and it varies in width from base to apex. The basilar membrane is most narrow and stiffer at the oval window, 100 micrometers. In contrast, the membrane is wider and more flexible at the apex, exhibiting a width of 500 micrometers. At low frequencies, the peak amplitude is closer to the apex near the helicotrema and then as the frequencies increase, the peak amplitude will move closer to the base. In the apex the stereocilia are twice as long as those at the base. The stereocilia are also more flexible at the apex than at the base. The creation of a mechanical resonance system is the net effect of this entire conversion of mechanical energy to mechanochemicoelectrical energy.

The cochlea is tonographically arranged, it exhibits a property termed "tuning of the cochlea" that is brought about through this tonographic representation. This property is found by the basilar membrane having differing tones stimulate different nerve endings. The vibrations of the hair cells are transposed to the bipolar neurons of the spiral ganglions within the modiulus of the cochlea. 90% of the fibers of these neurons will innervate the inner hair cells while the remaining 10% of the neurons will innervate the outer hair cells. The efferents of the CNS will also synapse on the afferent axons that innervate the hair cells. The outer hair cells are able to contract the entire length of the cell body producing a mechanical change to the properties of the Organ of Corti. So, it is therefore possible that since the outer hair cells are innervated by the CNS efferents, these length changes may be under neural control. Inner hair cells detect sounds and stimulate most of the afferent fibers of the auditory nerve. The selective modulation properties of the outer hair cells combined with the ability to change the mechanical properties of the Organ of Corti may provide the brain with the ability to either tune in or tune out sounds. Spiral ganglion cells innervate only a single hair cell and the individual fibers of the auditory nerve respond to a particular frequency. Fibers that innervate the hair cells near the oval window at the base have a high frequency characteristic where the fibers near the apex will have characteristics of low frequency sounds.

Nerve fibers cannot fire with a fast enough repetition to follow a high pitch sound with a one action potential per sound wave theory. The firing of the afferent fibers will be limited to approximately 0.5 KHz due to the refractory period of the nerve. The upper ranges of hearing are known to extend to a frequency of 20 Hz. This property of hearing means that there must be another mechanism of firing other than the one to one theory. The temporal brain activity patterns of responses to a brief tone burst even at frequencies < 500 Hz is not instantaneous in its response. The low frequency tone use phase locking at frequencies below 400 Hz and speech signals are mainly under 400 Hz.

The spiral ganglion is made up of two types of bipolar neurons, sensory neurons. Type 1 cells constitute 90-95% of these cells. They demonstrate radial branches that have very few synapses, typically 1-2 inner hair cells. There are as many as 20 or more Type 1 radial fibers to converge on each inner hair cell. Because of this distribution of fibers, Type 1 cells have a very narrow range of auditory stimulation. Type 2 cells will traverse the Tunnel of Corti and will synapse with more than 10 outer hair cells. Type 2 cells are more sensitive to low intensity sounds. The frequency is encoded in the cochlear nerve by a position of the afferent along the cochlear spiral. The central auditory neurons are specialized cells. The physiologic properties of these cells provide them with a very unique function; they are able to preserve time and frequency information. The auditory nerve fibers in the 8th cranial nerve, the vestibulocochlear nerve terminate in the cochlear nucleus within the external aspect of the inferior cerebral peduncle. The cochlear nucleus is then divided into a dorsal and ventral subdivision. The ventral subdivision is further subdivided into the anteroventral and the posteroventral cochlear nuclei. Every fiber that will enter the nucleus will be seen to bifurcate with the ascending fibers projecting to the anteroventral cochlear nuclei and the descending fibers projecting to the posteroventral cochlear nuclei.

All of the fibers within the cochlear nerve will synapse within the cochlear nuclei. These fiber bundles include the trapezoid body, the acoustic stria, the lateral lemniscal, and the brachium of the inferior colliculus. The associated cell groups are the nuclei of the superior olivary complex and the trapezoid body, the lateral lemniscus and the inferior colliculus. The medial geniculate nucleus receives the auditory signals from the inferior colliculus and then relays them to the sublenticular limb of the internal capsule for further projection and termination in the auditory cortex.

These inputs will dessucate at a variety of levels in such a manner that the inputs will reach the system in one of two ways. The first way is through monoaural information that is routed to the contralateral side of the brain. The second way is through the binaural information inputs. These auditory dessucations, especially the level of the trapezoid body are just like the optic chiasm but have been referred to as the functional acoustic chaism. In the binaural system, the information is handled by a central pathway that will receive and then compare the impulses and project them to higher centers. Biaural pathways are performing the computations required to localize brief sounds. The factors that may affect the pathway will be the speed of the sound or the medium of transmission. This localization is accomplished through a comparison of the sound input delay from each side of the head as sound inputs. Axons of the cochlear nucleus will exit via three pathways. One pathway is the dorsal acoustic stria, the second being the intermediate acoustic stria and the final being the Trapezoid body. In comparison, the most important of the three is the Trapezoid body. The fibers that emerge from the Trapezoid body are seen to project and terminate in the superior olivary nucleus. The medial superior olive functions in localizing sound on the basis of the interaural time differences (ITD). These neurons are spindle shaped with one projection going medially, and the other being a laterally projecting dendrite. This dendrite will receive inputs from both the ipsilateral and contralateral cochlear nuclei. The lateral olive is responsible for the localization of sounds based upon the difference between sound intensities.

Axons from the superior olivary nucleus join both the crossed and the uncrossed fibers of the cochlear nucleus to form the lateral lemniscal pathway. These fibers travel through the lateral lemniscal nuclei on the way to the Commissure of Probst. Within this commissure, there is extensive crossing of the neural fibers. All of the fibers of the lateral lemniscal pathway will project and terminate in the inferior colliculus. Fibers that originate from the inferior colliculus will then project to the medial geniculate body of the thalamus, ipsilaterally. The medial geniculate body will have axons arise and project ipsilaterally to the primary auditory cortex of the superior temporal gyrus, also known as Broadmans area 41-42.

The cochlear nucleus is made from a complex set of cell groups on the lateral aspect of the medulla. These fibers are found lateral and dorsal to the restiform body near the pontomedullary junction. The ventral cochlear nucleus is seen to project in a rostral to dorsal arrangement. It is possible to be covered by the flocculus and the caudal fascicles of the middle cerebral peduncle. All of these auditory nerves will penetrate ipsilaterally and then bifurcate.

Nerve fibers entering the nuclei will bifurcate with some becoming the innervation for the cells of the anteroventral cochlear nucleus (AVCN) and others descending to become the cells innervating neurons posteroventral cochlear nucleus (PVCN) and the dorsal cochlear nuclei (DCN). There is variable crossing and uncrossing of the ascending fibers of this pathway as the fibers makes their way to the lower brain stem. The anterior portion of the ventral nucleus contains spherical and globular shaped Bushy cells. There is a near 1 to 1 relationship between the synaptic endings of the cochlear nerve and a bushy cell. The axons of the Bushy cell will then project into the trapezoid body. They are the central origin of the ascending channels that process binaural information. The ventral cochlear nucleus also contains multipolar cells that are sensitive to the pressure changes associated with the sound waves. They convert information on the direct monoaural pathway to the contralateral inferior colliculous about the intensities of the sound.

Octopus cells are another type of cell seen in the posterior portion of the ventral cochlear nucleus. The octopus cells histologically, are seen to exhibit the long unbranched dendrites. These cells will synapse in the contralateral ventral nucleus of the lateral lemniscal pathway. These fibers will in turn project on to the inferior colliculus. The function of this pathway is for the brief analysis of speech sounds. The dorsal nucleus has pyramidal cells with fusiform bodies, apical and basal dendrites. These are a major output of the dorsal cochlear nucleus. The fibers will continue and project on to the contralateral inferior colliculus.

The superior olivary complex is found within the tegmentum of the pons and has several subdivisions. The key here is that it is the first point where the outputs from the two ears converge. Structurally, differing subdivisions of this complex are involved in the differing aspects of processing of the auditory signals. This is especially true with binaural signal processing. The fibers of this complex will project on to the inferior colliculi of both sides via the lateral lemniscal pathway as well as to the lateral lemniscal nuclei themselves. The complex is also the source of the efferent projections back to the hair cells of the cochlea.

The medial superior olivary nucleus (MSO) is seen as a distinct vertical bar in the periolivary nuclei. It is the main nuclei in the human superior olivary nucleus. The axons here will travel to the Ipsilateral lateral lemniscus. From the lateral lemniscus the fibers will continue on projecting to synapse within the central nucleus of the inferior colliculus. It is the medial superior olivary nucleus that will determine the location of the auditory stimulus based on the interaural time differences. The lateral superior olivary nuclei is quite indistinct. The fibers of this cell collection create a lateral projection that will constitute an indirect binaural pathway from the superior olivary nucleus to the inferior colliculus.

The trapezoid body is a group of fibers that is seen to run ventrally to the superior olivary nucleus and it will intermingle with the fibers of the medial lemniscal pathway as it crosses midline. These fibers will terminate in the superior olivary nucleus. Some of the fibers will however, continue on as the projections to the contralateral lemniscal pathway. These afferents are also tonographically arranged. Those cells with a low frequency characteristic are found dorsally while those with high frequency characteristics are found to lie ventrally. In these neurons, the neurotransmitter is glutamate or aspartate will provide the excitatory function and Glycine is most likely the inhibitory neurotransmitter.

The lateral lemniscus contains second order axons from the cochlear nucei and third order neurons in the superior olive and fourth order neurons in the adjacent fields of the lateral lemniscus. The large ventral nucleus of the lateral lemniscus consists of cells that are scattered among the ascending fibers of the lateral lemniscus. The small dorsal nucleus of the lateral lemniscus is seen to be interspersed within the ascending fibers of the lateral lemniscus, caudal to the inferior colliculus. The inputs to the system are mainly from the superior olivary nucleus. The ascending projections from the dorsal nucleus will dessucate within the dorsal tegmental commissure. The projection fibers will terminate in the contralateral inferior colliculus. The function of this pathway is as an inhibitor not an excitatory pathway. The neurotransmitter in this pathway is GABA. Functionally, the pathway is used to convey binaural information while concurrently inhibiting the activity from the opposite hemisphere.

The inferior colliculus is seen as the caudal pair of protuberances that will make up the roof of the midbrain. It has a core of the central nucleus that is formed from the fibers of the lateral lemniscus. These fibers will be the major input to the inferior colliculus contralaterally. Surrounding the central nucleus is the pericentral dorsal nucleus and the paracentral nucleus. The cells of the paracentral nucleus will habitate rapidly with repetitive stimuli. Inputs are from the central nuleus and the cerebral cortex with non-auditory inputs from the spinal cord, the dorsal column nuclei and the superior colliculus. These neurons will in turn project to the medial geniculate body, the superior colliculus, the reticular formation, and the precerebellar nuclei. There are many inputs that project from the cochlear nuclear complex, superior olivary complex, nuclei of the lateral lemniscus and the opposite inferior colliculus. These inputs are of verbal and non verbal origins. All of the fibers from the ascending portion of the lateral lemniscus will synapse here. These fibers are very sensitive to small changes in the arrival time of a stimulus at the two ears or in small differences in the intensities of the interaural sounds. Structurally, it is tonographicaly arranged as has been previously discussed. It only sends axons centrally as far as the medial geniculate body. It does however receive descending projections from the auditory cortex. Outputs from the inferior colliculus will descend via the brachium projecting to the medial geniculate body of the thalamus. The majority of the projections are Ipsilateral with some of the projections being contralateral.

The medial geniculate body is the thalamic relay of auditory information. This is seen to lie at the lower caudal surface of the thalamus between the lateral geniculate body and the pulvinar. The medial geniculate body will send out projections to the auditory cortex. From the auditory cortex, projections will run out to return to the medial genicuate body in a circuit like manner. The ventral division will receive the inputs from the central nucleus of the inferior colliculus and then project on to the primary auditory cortex. Low frequencies are seen to activate laterally and the higher tones are found medially. The dorsal division will receive inputs from the pericentral nucleus of the inferior colliculus. Axons will project from the dorsal division on to the secondary auditory cortex. The function of this neural pathway is the ability to convey information about new experiences or movement. The medial division or the magnocellular division afferents are from the external nucleus of the inferior colliculus. It will project axons on to the association areas of the auditory cortex. From the auditory cortex, projections will then go to the parietal association areas of the amygdale, the putamen, and the pallidum. Therefore it is a part of the reticular activating system.

The auditory cortex, the primary auditory cortex, auditory association cortices are located in the dorsal aspect of the superior temporal lobe, which is the transverse Gyri of Heschel or Broadmans areas 41-42. The gyrus is found within the horizontal plane deep into the Sylvian fissure in the posterior temporal lobe. Perception of the auditory information is done within this set of tissue. Each auditory cortical area has complex afferent and efferent connections within the thalamus as well as auditory connections to the opposite hemisphere. This structure sets up a paradigm for the forced crossing of listening called dichotic listening. In dichotic listening, the right ear, left brain shows nonverbal advantage. This is evidenced by the posterior 1/3 of the superior temporal gyrus, Broadmans area 22 that shows auditory association on the left. This is the area of decoding aural verbal information and on the right side it shows a non verbal association. The right side is responsible for the spectral information of pitch and harmony.

Structurally, the auditory cortex layers are the layers 4, 5, and 6. Layer 4 is described as an input layer while layer 5 is the recurrent projection back to the medial geniculate body. Then layer 6 is the recurrent fibers that project back to the inferior colliculus. Additional structural arrangement is seen in the columnar arrangement of the auditory cortex. The binaural cells are found in the columns of suppression and summation. In the suppression column, the cells are responsive to single ear dominance. There are important callosal connections. Each hemisphere is concerned with localization of sound on the contralateral side of the body. In humans, the cerebral cortex is composed of functional areas called Broca's areas and Wernicke's areas. These areas are related to the perception of speech.

In addition to the parallel paths, the auditory system has extensive arrangements of feedback pathways. Some cells in the auditory cortex will send axons back to the medial geniculate body while others will project to the inferior colliculus. The inferior colliculus will in turn send projections to the cochlear nucleus as recurrent fibers. There are additional feedback loops as the cells near the superior olivary complex that makes up the olivocochlear bundle that will terminate on the either the hair cells directly or on the afferents that innervate them.

The primary auditory cortex is located within the transverse gyrus of Heschel, Broadmans area 41. This area is reciprocally innervated with the ventral division and area 42 with the dorsal division of the medial geniculate body. The corpus callosum provides the reciprocal connections with the corresponding areas of the opposite hemisphere. The auditory association cortex surrounds the primary auditory area. It is found in the posterior portion of the superior temporal gyrus. It is connected to the primary auditory cortex through the arcuate fasciculus. Wernicke's area is the speech receptive area and possible to see it as much as seven times greater in size on the left than in the right. The higher association areas of the auditory cortex will extend into the inferior parietal lobe. Baroca's area, Broadman's 44-45, are functionally for the expressive ability of speech and language. The major path that comes from these areas is the primary and association areas is in the arcuate fasciculus.

The descending pathways are seen in the olivocochlear bundle, a descending efferent system that arises in the group of cells within the periolivary nuclei and the superior olivary complex. The lateral olivocochlear efferent projections are seen to project to the ipsilateral inner hair cells and make axo-axonic synapses with the Type 1 spiral ganglion. The medial olivocochlear efferent projections have bilateral projections that are seen to terminate on the outer hair cells directly.

MEMORY

Memory is defined as the ability to alter behavior on the basis of experience. Memory is the ability to recall past events at the conscious level and even at the unconscious level. Habitation is the simplest form of earning. The neural stimulus is repeated several times. There is a subsequent decreasing sensitivity to the stimulus, until eventually the stimulus is ignored completely. This is a non associative form of learning. Associative learning is where the organism learns about a relationship of one stimulus to another. The classic example is the conditional reflex. A conditional reflex is a reflex that is elicited to stimulus that previously elicited no response. This is acquired by repeatedly pairing the stimulus with another stimulus that does not elicit the same response. If the conditional stimulus is presented often enough without the pairing of the intended response, the response will eventually die out. This is extinction or internal inhibition. If the conditional response is reinforced from time to time, the conditional reflex will become permanent. Operant conditioning is the situation where the subject is taught to perform a task in order to obtain a reward or punishment. Sensitization is the repeated exposure to a stimulus that will increase the response elicited. Intercortical transfer of learning is accomplished via the corpus callosum. Experimental evidence has demonstrated that it has the neural capacity to code for the information from one eye to be remembered by the other visual field. This transfer of information is done through the commissures. The posterior commissure is responsible for the transfer of visual information. The anterior commissure is responsible for the transfer of auditory information and somatesthetic information.

Memory is subdivided into nondeclarative or reflexive memory and declarative memory. Nondeclarative memory is classical conditioning, skills and unconscious memory. Declarative memory is conscious recall of events. This type of memory can be converted to nondeclarative memory through repetition. New or facilitated pathways are called memory traces. It is these trace patterns that can be activated by the thinking mind and re-integrated as actual memories. Thoughts or consciousness or memories are the result of the stimulation of many parts of the brain. This activity involves the integration of the cerebral cortex, the thalamic lobes, the limbic regions and the reticular formation. It is the stimulation sequence of the limbic—thalamic—reticular—formation that will determine the specific nature of the thought. Memory has many subdivisions that have been defined. Destruction of a large part of the cerebral cortex does not prevent a person from having thoughts but it will decrease the person's state of awareness.

Short term memory is the reproduction or recognition or recall of materiel within a period of 30 seconds or less. This time period may be extended to minutes as there may be continued neural activity that is secondary to the signals traveling around and around in a circuit of reverberating neuronal activity that is the memory trace. The mechanism for this process is thought to be the actual circuit of reverberating neurons and presynaptic facilitation—inhibition and it may be due to the synaptic potentiation that can enhance the synaptic conductivity. This increased conductivity is due in part to the increased calcium levels in the presynaptic cell. Lesions to this system are possible to be very devastating. If the lesion is on the right hemisphere of the brain, the resultant defect will produce visual defects while defects to the left hemisphere will produce auditory problems. Short term memory is an immediate type of memory. It is also called working memory, primary memory, or buffer memory. The key here is the amount of information that is able to be stored is very small, approximately 5-9 bytes. Smell and emotion are underlying factors in the conversion of memory from short term memory traces to long term memory traces. Smell conveys information via cranial nerve I to the hippocampus and as the hippocampus is seen to play a role in the recall of emotions. Prior to the age of 3-5 years, the only memories that are committed to long term memory will be those of trauma or olfaction. In instances where the information is important, such as pain or pleasure, the brain has an automatic capacity for enhancing and storing the memory traces. This is the function of the process of facilitation of the synaptic properties.

The process of memory sensitization is where special regions of the basal limbic regions are responsible for the determination if the information is important enough to be stored or not. It then makes a subconscious decision to store the trace as a memory or to suppress the information. Descriptions of memory are recent memory being memory traces that are from the past hours or even days. Recent past memories are those that are of events from the past few months. Episodic memory is describes as the memory of special events. Semantic memory is a specific knowledge of facts, but not idiot savant. Implicit memory is the memory of skill sets like driving. This memory type does not alter with increasing age. Repeated living of the event is going to increase the probabilities that the memory will be converted to permanent memory traces. Storage is the key to good memory to good memory. If you relate the event to something already integrated in the permanent memory trace as well.

Intermediate long term memory is something that may last for minutes to several weeks. It will eventually be lost unless the memory traces are converted to long term permanent memories. In long term memories there is an actual change in the neural circuitry. These changes are not chemical changes they are real structural circuitry changes. These changes are synaptic changes, where the synapse will reconstruct itself. Te synapse will be more sensitive to transmission of impulses via the increased number of vesicles within the active zone to be released presynaptically. Additionally, there is an associated increase in the number of vesicles released such that the actual number of vesicles released may double. In this process, the actual length of the axons and dendrites are able to increase to accommodate the actual synaptic changes.

The hippocampus plays a role in the function of memory storage. The hippocampus is the most medial aspect of the temporal lobe and it folds first medially up into the lower surface of the ventricles. Experimental evidence demonstrates that excision of the hippocampus will elicit memories that would be committed after its removal. The excision of the hippocampus will not however, adversely affect those memories established prior to excision. The hippocampus is also the most important path for the outputs from the limbic system, those of reward and punishment. The hippocampus works with the dorsal medial nucleus of the thalamus have proven to be intricate in the ability of decision making processes for the conversion of memory traces to be retained and which memory traces are to be suppressed. This decision is based on the reward and punishment center of the limbic center. The thalamus is important in the search for memory within the system of recall.

Consolidation of memory is something that must be done if memories are to be stored and converted. For short term memory to be converted to long term memory it must first be consolidated. This is the process if initiating a chemical, physical and anatomic change in the synapse itself in preparation for the actual conversion. This process requires approximately 5-10 minutes for the minimal amount of consolidation and as much as 1 hour for maximal consolidation to occur. If there is a strong impression to go along with the memory trace that is relayed to the brain, but then if this activity is followed by increased electrical activity that is obtrusive, the memory will not be stored. If the increased electrical activity is delayed for a little as 10 minutes, the information will be stored as a memory trace. If the activity is delayed for one hour, the activity will have time to be converted to a long term memory.

Rehearsal of memory is when there is a closed circuit of electrical activity that accelerates the memory trace conversion into long term memory. This phenomenon is seen if the activity is interesting to the individual. If they deem the activity interesting the memory will be easily and rapidly converted to long term permanent memory. One important feature of consolidation is that memories are coded into different classes of information. The brain constantly scans old memories and compares them with new ones. If the new memories are similar to the old ones, the new memories will be more easily encoded than those that are unfamiliar. The rationale for this ease of encoding will be seen as the memory traces will be stored in direct association with the old ones. This is the reason for the details of certain events being confused when recalling certain events.

The primary sensory areas will detect specific sensations such as visual, auditory and somatic. These sensations are then relayed to the higher cortical centers. Secondary association center makes sense of the information that has been sent from the primary areas. The secondary association areas are in close proximity to the primary association areas. The secondary association areas are responsible for the interpretation of shape, texture, color, light intensity, direction, angles, sounds, tones and the beginning of the auditory signals.

The association areas are the parieto-occipitotemporal, the prefrontal and the limbic regions. The parieto-occipitotemporal area is also the somatosensory cortex in the anterior aspect and the visual cortex in the posterior cortex and laterally, the auditory cortex is seen. The areas adjacent and surrounding them are the integrative areas. Wernicke's area is the area for the language comprehension. It is found to lie posterior to the auditory cortex in the posterior aspect of the superior gyrus of the temporal lobe. It is thought by many persons to be the most important area for higher learning since most aspects of higher learning are language comprehension based. The initial process of visual language comes from the angular gyrus of the occipital lobe. This area feeds visual data by the words read from print to Wernicke's area. The naming of the objects is done via learned names from hearing stimuli. The brains account of the actual physical nature of the object is accomplished by the visual input.

Prefrontal areas work closely with the motor cortex for the planning of complex motor patterns. The output of this area is the caudate portion of the basal ganglia to the thalamus feedback system. This provides sequential and parallel components of movement stimulation. This is thought to be essential for the long term memory process to become ingrained. This process is called the elaboration of thought. The elaboration of thought is the increase in the depth and the abstractness if different thoughts are put together from multiple sources of information. The prefrontal areas are divided into separate areas for the storage of different types of memories. This means that there may be one region for the storage of object data and another for storage of movements.

Baroca's area is the area of neural circuitry of word formation. It is seen to lie within the posterolateral prefrontal cortex and partially in the premotor area. This area is responsible for the motor plans of facial expression of individual words or short phrases as well as the initiation and execution of those words and phrases. The interpretative function of the posterior superior temporal lobe, or Wernicke's area is the source of the somatic, auditory association, and visual information. This area is especially highly developed on the left side. It has the greatest single role of ant part of the cerebral cortex in the higher brain levels we call intelligence. Higher intellectual functions of the prefrontal cortex association areas show that destruction of the language comprehension are of the posterior superior temporal lobe, Wernicke's area, and the adjacent angular gyrus of the dominant hemisphere will have more devastating effects on intellect than damage to the prefrontal areas. Remember that the dominant hemisphere is the left and that this area may be up to 50% larger than the like on the right side. The corpus callosum and the anterior commissure functions to make available data stored in one hemisphere to the appropriate areas of the opposite hemisphere. The amygdala is also connected via the anterior commissure. Another function of the corpus callosum and the anterior commissure is the transfer of thoughts and memories between the two hemispheres. The exception to this functional role is the anterior temporal lobes. This is closely associated with both the primary hearing area of the temporal lobe and the secondary hearing center. It is thought the Wernicke's area is able to call for the more complicated memory patterns that involve more than one sensory modality, even though most of the memory patterns are stored elsewhere. The Limbic association region is found in the anterior pole of the temporal lobe. It is responsible for the regulation of behavior, emotions, and motivation of the individual. This includes a complex set of neuronal structures on the midbasal regions of the brain. It is the emotional drive of this region that sets the other regions in action.

Nerve signals in the brain stem activate the cerebral cortex in one of two ways. Either by direct stimulation of the background level activity in wide areas of the brain or by activation of neurohormonal systems. The control of the cerebral activity by continuous excitation signals from the brain stem is achieved through the reticular formation being the central driving force. The reticular formation is the driving force for the excitatory area called the bulboreticular facilitory area. This is found on the reticular substance of the pons and the mesencepheon. This area sends signals up to the thalamus and then projections on to the remainder of the cerebral cortex. The signals that are sent to the thalamus are of two types, one is a rapidly transmitted action potential that is able to excite the cerebrum for milliseconds and the other is a signal that originates from the large number of neurons spread throughout the brain stem reticular formation's excitatory area. The vast majority of the signals will project to the thalamus through the intralaminar nuclei. There is a particular property of these neurons in that they have the ability to have a delayed build up of the action potentials. The excitation of the brain stem excitatory area is done via the peripheral sensory signals. The levels of the activity of the brain stem excitatory area as well as the entire brain will be determined by the sensory signals sent through by the peripheral system. There are recurrent paths from the buboreticular excitatory area to the cortex. This same system has a return recurrent pathway. This means that when the cerebral cortex is activated by thought or motor processes, there will be signals that will go back to the brain stem excitatory area that will in turn activate additional excitatory signals to the cerebral cortex. The thalamus is the distribution center that controls activity in specific regions of the cortex. The signals that reverberate between the cortex and the thalamus are thought to assist in the establishment of the long term memories.

The reticular inhibitory areas of the lower medulla, the ventral and the medial medulla are responsible for the decreased activity of the reticular excitatory system. Through this mechanism, the stimulation is able to decrease the tonic muscle activity. This system uses serotoninergic neurons. This is one possible explanation for the increased functional activity with TBI and music therapy.

The behavioral functions of the hypothalamus laterally, elicit increased thirst and increased general metabolic activity. Stimulation of the ventromedial area has the exact opposite effects in thirst and metabolism. Stimulation of the thin paraventricular zone adjacent to the 3rd ventricle will elicit fear and punishment reactions. If the anterior posterior hypothalamus is stimulated, there is increased sex drive.

CHAPTER 23

NEUROANATOMY

A) Medulla Oblongata
   a. Most caudal portion of the brain
   b. Consists of
      i. Neurons that perform functions with the medulla
      ii. Ascending & descending tracts that pass through
   c. Contains the nuclei of the glossopharyngeal CN IX, vagas (CN X), hypoglossal (CN XII) as well as portions of the nuclei for the trigeminal, vestibulocochlear, spinal accessory
   d. Contains relay centers essential for the regulation of respiration, HR rate and visceral functions

B) Pons & Cerebellum
   a. Embryologically, origination is from the same part of the neural tube.
   b. As adult, pons is part of the brainstem.
   c. Cerebellum is suprasegmental, as it is located dorsal to the brainstem.

d. Pons contains: both ascending & descending tracts,
    i. Nuclei of the abducens, facial, portions of the trigeminal and vestibulocochlear,
    ii. Ventral portion are the relay neurons that connect the cortex and the cerebellum
e. Cerebellum is considered as part of the motor system. Coordinates activity of individual muscle groups to produce smooth coordinated movements.

C) Midbrain
  a. Link between the brainstem and the forebrain.
  b. Ascending and descending tracts must traverse the midbrain
  c. Contains the nuclei for
    i. Occulomotor
    ii. Trochlear
    iii. Part of the trigeminal
    iv. Visual & auditory reflex pathways, motor function, transmission of pain & visceral functions

D) Thalamus
  a. Found within the forebrain
  b. Consists of the hypothalamus, subthalamus, epithalamus and the dorsal thalamus, the ventral thalamus
  c. Located rostral to the midbrain.
  d. All sensory information except olfaction passes through the thalamus to the cortex

E) Hypothalamus
  a. Functions in sexual behavior, feeding, hormonal output of the pituitary gland, body temperature
  b. Influences visceral centers in the brainstem and the spinal cord.

F) Cerebral hemispheres
  a. Each is divided into 3 major subdivisions. Many association areas essential for analysis and cognitive thought processing.
    i. Cortex—layer of neuronal cell bodies 0.5 cm thick

1. Covers the entire surface of the hemisphere
2. Indentations are called sulci
3. Elevations are called gyri

ii. Subcortical white matter-myelinated axons that carry information to and from the cortex

1. Largest and most organized portion of the subcortical white matter is the internal capsule

iii. Basal ganglia—involved in motor function

G) Axons

a. Arise from the cell body at the axonal hillock. The proximal portion of the axon adjacent to the axonal hillock is the initial segment
b. Cytoplasm of the axon contains lots of microtubules and microfilaments
c. Typically devoid of ribosomes
d. In the CNS, often terminate in fine branches called terminal arbors.
e. If the axon terminal is capped with a small boutton it is called a terminal boutton, or if the axon only contains swelling, then the swellings are called varicosities and offer a point of information transfer. If the bouttons are found along the axon then they are termed boutton en passant.

H) Axonal Transport

a. From the cell body to the terminals is termed anterograde or orthograde.

i. Anterograde axonal transport fast—400 mm/day using protein called kinesin, an ATPase will move macromolecules & mitochondria

ii. Anterograde axonal transport slow—carries structural and metabolic components. Allows the neuron to respond to things like growth factors.

b. From the terminals to the cell body is termed retrograde and utilizes the protein dyenin.

I) Spinal cord—participates in 4 vital functions
   a. Receives primary sensory input from the receptors as somatosensory information and viscerosensory information.
   b. Contains the somatic motor neurons that innervate striated muscle and the visceral motor neurons.
   c. Somatosensory fibers enter the spinal cord and influence the ventral horn motor neurons either directly or indirectly through interneurons. The activated motor neurons in turn produce rapid involuntary contractions of skeletal muscle. The sensory fiber, the associated motor neuron, and the resultant involuntary movement are called the spinal reflex.
   d. Contains the descending fibers that influence the activity of the spinal neurons. These fibers originate in the cerebral cortex or brainstem.

J) Spinal cord structure—butterfly shaped central area of gray matter (neuron cell bodies) surrounded by white matter (myelinated fibers) with a central core called the central canal
   a. Extends from the foramen magnum to the level of L1-2
   b. Has a cervical enlargement (C4-T1) and a lumbosacral enlargement (L1-S2)
   c. Posterior median sulcus—separates the dorsal portion of the cord into two halves and contains a delicate layer of pia (posterior median septum). The posteriolateral sulcus runs the full length of the cord represents the entry point of the dorsal (sensory) root fibers. It is also called the dorsal root entry zone.
   d. On the ventrolateral surface, of the spinal cord, the anterolateral sulcus is the exit point for the ventral root.
   e. Anterior median fissure divides the ventral part of the cord into two halves. The fissure contains the delicate strands of pia and the sulcal branches of the anterior spinal artery.

K) Spinal meminges
   a. Caudal end of the cord it anchored to the coccyx by the filum terminal externum.

Pathways and tracts of the spinal cord

1. Spinal cord white matter—consists of
   A) long ascending and descending fibers & tracts. Motor activities and pain transmission
   B) propriospinal fibers that project from on e spinal level to another. Therefore interspinal reflexes

2. Ascending tracts
   A) dorsal column is made up of the gracile & cuneate fasciculi. These fibers are heavily myelinated primarily sensory fibers that convey proprioception, tactile, vibratory senses from the ipsilateral side. The gracile fasciculus originates in the sacral, lumbar and thoracic (below T6). The cuneate fasciculus originates from the upper thoracic (above T6) and cervical levels. Injury produces ipsilateral loss of proprioception, discriminative sensation, vibratory sense below the level of the lesion.
   B) the posterior(dorsal), spinocerebellar & anterior (ventral) spinocerebellar tracts are located in the lateral surface of the cord all meeting at the level of the denticulate ligament. Fibers of the former tract arise from clarkes nuclei in the lamina VII at T 1-T2 while the latter arise from lamina V & VIII and from the large ventral horn neurons called the spinal border cells, both at lumbosacral levels.
   C) in the ventrolateral area is the large bundle called the ALS—anterolateral system. This is the encompassing of the white matter that is classically divided into the anterior & lateral spinothalamic tracts. ALS contains the, spinomesencephalic (spinotectal, spinoperiaqueductal), spinohypothalamic & spinoreticular fibers.
   The ALS originate mainly from the dorsal horn but some arise from the ventral horn. The fibers of the ALS cross in the ventral white commissure ascending one or two levels as they do so. ALS fibers convey nocioception, thermal, and touch data. Injury results in loss of pain, temp, cruder touch on contralateral side beginning 1-2 levels below the lesion.

D) spinocervicothalamic tract—originate in lamina III-VIII but mainly IV. And ascend in the dorsal part of the lateral funiculus to terminate in the lateral cervical nucleus at C 1-C3. postsynaptic dorsal column fibers originate in the lamina III-VIII but mainly IV and ascend ipsilaterally in the dorsal columns.
E) spino-olivary
F) spinovestibular
G) spinoreticular

3. Descending tracts—the lateral fascicles contains the lateral corticospinal and the rubrospinal tracts, the anterior funiculus, the reticulospinal, vestibulospinal tracts, The medial longitudinal fasciculus (MLF). The MLF is composed of: medial vestibulospinal fibers, tectospinal fibers and interstitiospinal fibers (of the interstitial nucleus of the rostral midbrain and some reticulospinal fibers) the tectospinal and the vestibulospinal fibers are contained in the cervical cord.
The vestibulospinal tracts are made of the medial and the lateral. The lateral vestibulospinal fibers originate from the lateral vestibular nucleus and the medial from the medial vestibular nucleus.
A) reticulospinal fibers—originate in the medullary reticular formation. At spinal levels the fibers are uncrossed
B) fastigiospinal fibers—originate in the fastigial nucleus of the cerebellum. These fibers are crossed. Function is to maintain posture, therefore these fibers tend to excite extensor motor neurons and inhibit flexor motor neurons.
C) raphespinal fibers—originate in the rap he nuclei of the brain stem. Descend bilaterally in the dorsal areas of the lateral funiculus. Function is modulate nocioceptive information at the spinal levels.
D) hypothalamospinal fibers—originate in the hypothalamus a nd descend through the lateral brainstem. Function is to influence the GVE motor neurons. Lesions in the brainstem or the spinal cord that effect this will produce Horner's syndrome—ptosis, miosis, anhidrosis & enopthalamos.
E) corticospinal tracts—originate in the cerebral cortex and descend through the brainstem. At the medulla—spinal level the majority

of the fibers will cross to form the lateral corticospinal tract. These fibers will stimulate the flexor motor neurons and inhibit the extensor motor neurons. These fibers are somatotopically arranged. The fibers that originate from the leg areas of the cortex are found laterally, where the fibers that originate from the areas representing the arms are medially located. Important function is the influence of the fine motor function of the distal musculature. Therefore, lesion of a portion of the cord will elicit paralysis of the arm and leg on the same side as the lesion. Some will remain uncrossed as the anterior corticospinal tract.

F) rubrospinal fibers—originate in the red nucleus of the midbrain and cross at that level, descend in the spinal cord with the fibers of the lateral corticospinal tract. Stimulate mainly the flexor motor neurons and inhibit the extensor motor neurons. (together with the lateral corticospinal tract)

SPINAL CORD

1. Spinal cord participates in 4 functions

A. Receives primary sensory input from the receptors in the skin, skeletal mm, and tendons (somatosensory fibers) as well as receptors in the thoracic, abdominal and pelvic viscera (viscerosensory) through multi synaptic relays in the spinal cord
B. SC contains somatic motor neurons that innervate striated MM

Frontal lobe—from frontal pole to the central sulcus.

A) consists of pre central gurus,
premotor cortex,
supplementary motor cortex,
frontal eye field,
motor speech area (Broca's area)
prefrontal cortex

Occipital lobe—posterior, to the temporal lobe while inferior to the parietal lobe

A) V1—primary visual cortex
V2—secondary visual cortex
V3—third visual cortex

Parietal lobe—superior to the occipital lobe & the temporal lobe while separated from the frontal lobe by the central sulcus

A) V5 / hMT
Post central gurus
Primary somatosensory cortex
Secondary somatosensory cortex
Supramarginal gurus
Angular gyrus

Temporal lobe—inferior to the lateral sulcus

A) superior temporal gyrus
Middle temporal gyrus
Inferior temporal gyrus
V4
Auditory tract
Primary auditory cortex
Secondary auditory cortex

Gyri

Cinglulate gyrus—posterior region—Braodmann area 29, 26, 30, 22, 31

Anterior region Broadmann area 33, 24, 25, 32

Found on the medial wall below the frontal & parietal lobe immediately superior to the callosum yet inferior to the cingulate sulcus

On the posterior aspect it passes the splenum of the corpus callosum. To turn inferiorly as the narrow isthmus of the cingulate gyrus the cingulate cortex and parahippocampal gyrus, together with the olfactory bulb and tract, and certain other small cortical areas, are often referred to separately as the limbic lobe (from limbus = border)

Important part of the limbic system, coordinates sensory input with emotional output. It receives input from the anterior nucleus of the thalamus and the neocortex. It projects to the entorhinal cortex via the cingluum

Cuneus—wedged shaped area on the medial surface between the parietooccipital and calcerine sulcus
Secondary visual areas dorsal V2 & V3

Gyrus Rectus—found on the basal portion of the frontal lobe running parallel to the olfactory tact. Found between the gyrus rectus and the orbital gyri is the olfactory sulcus
Functions in connectivity

Inferior Frontal Gryus—compromises about 1/3 of the frontal lobe, running. Orthogonal to the pre central sulcus and the lateral sulcus. It is visibly divided into three parts with the most anterior portion being the orbital portion and the most posterior portion being the opercular part. (forms the frontal operculum). Located between is the wedge shaped triangular portion.
Functions in connectivity Baroca's area is located within the opercular and the triangular parts of the left hemisphere and is important in the production of written and spoken language

Inferior Occipital Gyrus—found on the lateral surface of the occipital lobe
Functions in higher order processing of visual information

Inferior Parietal lobe—located with. The lateral surface inferior to the intraparietal sulcus, and composed of the supra marginal gyrus (this is the end of the lateral sulcus) and the angular gyrus(the end of the superior temporal sulcus)
Function s in connectivity within the left hemisphere it is known to be involved in the comprehension of language and the numerical processing

Inferior Temporal Gyrus—it is a continuation from the lateral to the inferior surface of the temporal lobe and it separates the medial frontal gyrus and the inferior frontal gyrus.
Functions in connectivity

Insula—deep in the lateral sulcus and is concealed by portions of the frontal, parietal and temporal lobes
It processes convergent information to produce emotionally relevant context for sensory experience such as disgust and feelings of being uneasy. Anatomically, there is distinction of function with the anterior insole being involved in the olfactory, gustatory, viceroautonomic, and limbic function. The posterior insular is related to more auditory and somesthetic—skeletomotor function. H been demonstrated by PET scan to be involved in the experience of pain. Therefore, it is thought to play a role in the fear avoidance of painful stimuli.

Lateral Occipito-temporal gyrus—also called the fusiform gyrus. It is found partially within the occipital lobe and partially within the temporal lobe and runs parallel to the parahippocampah gyrus
Functions in connectivity and higher order processing of visual information color processing and facial recognition (fusiform face area)

Lingual gyrus—found within the occipital lobe.
Functions in the early processing of visual information (V1, V2, V3) as well as higher processing of visual information and complex aspects of learning and memory.

Medial Occipitotemporal gyrus—is found within bothe e occipital and the temporal lobe, mostly in the temporal lobe, and contains the lingual gyrus, the parahippocampah gyrus and the entorhinal cortex.
Functions in the higher processing of visual information, the processing of places and houses as well as complex aspects of learning and memory.

Middle frontal gyrus—found within the frontal lobe and runs orthogonal to the pre central gyrus between the superior and inferior frontal gyrus.

Functions in the working memory, attention, planning control aspects of he brain as well as receiving and sending widespread connections wih higher cognitive functioning.

Middle Occipital Gyrus—contains the lateral occipital gyrus. Found between the superior and the inferior occipital gyrus
Functions in visual interpretation

Middle Temporal Gyrus—this is found in the lower region of the lateral surface of the Temporal lobe. It is serrated from the inferior temporal gyrus by the inferior temporal sulcus.

Orbital gyri—inferior (orbital) surface of the frontal lobe above the orbit

Parahippocampal gyrus—this is located on the medial side of the temporal lobe and is part of the limbic system and it contains part of the peri and enthorhinal cortex
Functions in the complex aspects of learning and memory, processes places.

Post central gyrus—contains the Broadmann's area BA3, BA2, and BA1. This is found as prominent structure as the most anterior surface area of the parietal lobe and it separates the central and the post central sulcus
Functions in the somatosensory organization (homunculus) SI, and BA2.

Precentral gyrus—contains Broadmann's area B4
Locatedin the frontal lobe anterior to the central sulcus
Functions in connectivity within th eprimary motor cortex M1

Precuneus—located in the lower medial surface of the parietal lobe
Functions in connectivity

Superior Frontal Gyrus—found superior to the frontal lobe and runs orthogonal to the pre central sulcus. It extends from the superior frontal sulcus (lateral surface) to the cingulate sulcus (medial surface). This is not strictly a gyrus but rather a region that constitutes about 1/3 of the frontal lobe

Functions in connectivity within the premotor area, it is thought to be related to the initiation of voluntary movements. Eye movement control and the frontal eye field. (FEF)

Superior Occipital Gyrus—found on the upper portion of the lateral surface of the occipital lobe.

Functions in the visual interpretations

Superior Parietal Lobe—contains planum polare, transverse gyri, planum temporal, temporal operculum.

It is found on the upper part of the lateral surface of the temporal lobe between the lateral sulcus and the superior temporal sulcus. It is bounded posteriorly by an imaginary line drawn from the pre occipital notch to the posterior end of the lateral sulcus.

Functions in the processing of auditory information and the identification of the location of sound. Connections with The primary auditory cortex A1 about the same as with the BA 41 and BA 42. The primary auditory cortex extends into the lateral sulcus as the transverse temporal gyri (Heschel's gyri). The auditory areas are arranged tonographically and as such are important in speech (Werneke's area BA 22p). This area is also involved in he cross modal integration of visual and auditory information.

Sulci

Calcerine sulcus—also known as the striate sulcus.

It is found separating the pre cuneus from the gyrus lingualis

The function of this sulci is in the primary visual cortex V1, to receive visual signals from the retina via the lateral geniculate nucleus (LGN). This is arranged retinotopically as a map of the visual field. This area projects to higher visual areas in the extra striate cortex.

Central Sulcus—also known as the Rolandic fissure or the fissure of Rolando.

The posterior bank of tissue is the primary somatosensory cortex while the anterior bank of tissue is the motor cortex or the homunculus. This area receives the signals from the premotor cortex and sends axons down the spinal cord.

Cingulate Sulcus—it is the posterior region which contains broadmann's areas 26, 29, 30, 22, 31.

The location of this is on the medial wall of the frontal and the parietal lobe inferior to the superior frontal gyrus and superior to the cingulate gyrus.

The function of the sulcus is to coordinate sensory input with emotion, conflict monitoring as part of the control system, and it receives and sends widespread connections as part of the control network

Collateral sulcus—is also called the occipitotemporal sulcus.

This is located partially in the occipital lobe and the temporal lobe and separates the lateral occipitaotemporal gyrus and the medial occipital gyrus.

Function is in the high level visual areas, including the fusiform face area and receives input from early and mid level visual areas.

Inferior frontal sulcus-

Inferior frontal lobe, runs orthogonal to the pre central sulcus as it separates the medial frontal gyrus from the inferior frontal gyrus.

It functions in work memory, attention, control, and planning. It receives and sends connections as a portion of the higher cognitive function network.

Inferior temporal sulcus—location is in the temporal lobe as it separates the medial gyrus from the inferior temporal gyrus

It functions in the cross interpretation of mutlit input data, visual and auditory information, therefore it receives information from all the sensory areas.

Intraparietal sulcus—found to run posteriorly from the post central sulcus to the occipital lobe as it separates the inferior parietal lobes.
It functions in the spatial processing of spatio-motor data. It revives connections from the visual and the premotor centers

Lateral occipital sulcus—found within the lateral occipital lobe.
If function sin the visual cortex

Lateral sulcus—AKA the Sylvian fissure, located within the inferior end of the lateral surface of the frontal and parietal lobes and surrounded at the posterior end by the supra marginal gyrus.

Lunate sulcus—found in the lateral occipital lobe
Functions in visual interpretations

Occipitotemporal sulcus—located partially in the temporal and occipital lobes. It is seen to separate the medial ocipitotemporal gyrus and the lateral occipitotemporal gyrus.
Functions in the reciept of visual inputs from early to the mid level visual areas.

Olfactory sulcus—located on the inferior (orbital) surface of the frontal lobe between the orbital gyri and the gyrus rectus
Function is in olfaction

Orbital sulci—found within the inferior (orbital) surface of the frontal lobe but superior to the orbita.
Functions in transmission of the visual inputs

Parietooccipital sulcus—this is the prominent landmark on the medial aspect of the brain as it separates the occipital and the parietal lobe.

Post central sulcus—found posterior to the post central gyrus
Functions with the somatosensory cortex as it receives inputs from the primary somatosensory cortex (central sulcus, post central gyrus)

Precentral sulcus—anterior to the pre central gyrus but posterior to the frontal lobe
Functions with the premotor cortex as it projects mainly to the primary motor Cortex M1

Subparietal sulcus—found in the medial parietal lobe.

Superior frontal sulcus—locoed in the superior frontal lobe and runs orthogonally to the pre central sulcus as it separates the superior frontal gyrus and the medial frontal gyrus
Function sin the premotor areas

Superior Temporal Sulcus—located in the temporal lobe as it separates the medial temporal gyrus from the superior temporal gyrus
Function is the integration of the visual and auditory information as it will revise information from the sensory areas.

Transverse Occipital Sulcus—found on the lateral surface of the occipital lobe.

Broadmann's area's

BA 1—post central gyrus & anterior parietal pole.
Function is with the medial somatosensory cortex with basic somatosensory functions, working together with BA 2& BA 3contains the somatosensory homunculus

BA 2—post central gyrus and the anterior parietal lobe.
Functions in Caudal region of the somatosensory cortex. Working with BA 1 forms the somatosensory homunculus.

BA3—found in the post central gyrus and the anterior parietal lobe.
Functions with the rostral region of the somatosensory cortex for basic somatosensory functions. Together with BA1 and BA 2 contain the somatosensory homunculus.

BA4—it is the primary motor cortex. Locate within the precentral gyrus and anterior to the central sulcus.
Functions as the home of the motor homunculus, and as such is regulator fo the voluntary motor movements. It is connected to BA 6anteriorly and BA 1, BA2 and BA 3 posteriorly. There are also connections to the lateral ventral nucleus o the thalamus.

BA 5—this is found within the Parietal lobe at the prepyriform cortex.
Functions as part of the secondary somatosensory cortex in conjunction with BA 7.

BA 6—located within the Frontal lobe at the post central gyrus.
Functions in conjunction with BA 8 to form the premotor cortex, and in sensory guidance of motion and the control of proximal trunk and proximal MM.

BA 7—this is found within the parietal cortex posterior to the somatosensory cortex but superior to the visual cortex.
Function is in the integration of visual and motor data.

BA 8—this is located within tht frontal lobe.
Function is in the planning of movement within the pre motor cortex.

BA 9—this is located within the frontal lobe.
Function is in conjunction with BA 10 & 11 to make up the prefrontal cortex and to perform executive functions and cognitive control

BA 10—this is found in the frontal lobe in the rostral region of the superior frontal gyrus
Function with BA9& 11 to make up the prefrontal cortex, executive functions and cognitive control

BA 11—found in the medial part of the ventral surface of the frontal lobe, specifically the orbitofrontal cortex.
Function with BA 9& 10 to make up the prefrontal cortex. Executive functions and cognitive control

BA 17—AKA primary visual cortex, the striate cortex, V1
Located with the medial part of the occipital lobe.
Functions in the initial processing of visual information, organization is in ocular dominance columns, center of the fovea is represented at the occipital pole thus there is retinotopic organization with the larger representation of objects in the fovea. This also receives inputs from the lateral geniculate nucleus.

BA 18—AKA secondary visual cortex, V2, extra striate cortex
Located in the occipital pole and includes portions of the cuneas, lingual gyrus and the lateral occipital gyrus. This is considered as part of the extra striate cortex
Functions in visual processing

BA 19 found within the occipital lobe
Functions in visual processing and forms the extra striate visual cortex with BA 18

BA 20—is found within the inferior temporal lobe
Functions in hier level object representation, considered to be the visual ventral stream

BA 21-located within the lateral temporal lobe superior to BA 20 but inferior to BA 40 & BA 41. Found within the middle temporal gyrus
Functions in language and auditory processing

BA 22—located in the temporal lobe
Functions in the connectivity of the posterior Wernickie's area so assists in language comprehension

BA 23—located in the occipital lobe at the posterior portion of the cingulate cortex. Caudally it is bound by the occipital—parietal sulcus
Functions as part of the limbic system and is connected with the amygdyla, hippocampus, and the orbit-frontal cortex, so involved in the emotional display

BA 24—found in the ventral section of the cingulate cortex
Functions as part of the limbic system and is connected with the hippocampus, amygdala, so involved in emotional expression

BA 26—located in the retrospinal region. Specifically in the isthmus of the cingulate gyrus
Functions in the memory system, recall of episodic events

BA 27—located in the rostral aspect of the parahippocampal gyrus
Functions in memory trace development

BA 28—found in the medial aspect of the temporal lobe, the entorhinal area, adjacent to the subcortical hippocampus
Functions in the formation of memory traces.

BA 29—found in the retrosplenial regions and the isthmus of the cingulate gyrus.
Functions in the formation of memory traces and the recall of episodic events

BA—30 found in the retrosplenial regions and the isthmus of the cingulate gyrus.
Functions in the formation of memory traces and the recall of episodic events

BA 31—found in the isthmus of the cingulate gyrus
Functions in the processing of emotions and recognition

BA 32—found within the parietal lobe in the dorsal anterior cingulate
Functions in the decision making processes

BA 33—found within the anterior cingulate gyrus in the callosal sulcus
Functions in the decision making processes

BA 37—located in the temporal lobe the caudal portion of the fusiform gyrus and the inferior temporal gyrus

Functions in the multiple-modal integration and higher order object and facial recognition

BA 38—found within the temporal lobe the rostral section of the temporal gyrus and the middle temporal gyrus
Functions in the processing of memory and emotional association

BA 39—found within the parietal lobe corresponding with the angular gyrus
Function in semantic processing

BA 40—located in he parietal cortex in the area of the supra marginal gyrus at the posterior aspect of the lateral fissure and the superior aspect of the Sylvian fissure
Functions in secondary somatosensory representation and discrimination tasks

BA 41—AKA: Primary auditory cortex, found within the temporal lobe and the anterior transverse temporal gyrus the lateral sulcus
Functions in early processing of auditory data, this is topographically organized with the lower frequencies located more rostrally and lateral, while the higher frequencies more caudal and medial

BA 42—AKA: Primary auditory cortex, found within the temporal lobe and the anterior transverse temporal gyrus the lateral sulcus
Functions in early processing of auditory data, this is topographically organized with the lower frequencies located more rostrally and lateral, while the higher frequencies more caudal and medial

BA 44—AKA: Broca's area, Found in the inferior frontal lobe
Function is in the production of language

BA 45—found in the frontal cortex, specifically the Pars triangular of the inferior frontal gyrus. This borders with the insole in the lateral sulcus
Functions in the semantic tasking of word generation

BA 46—found in the frontal lobe, the middle frontal gyrus and parts of the dorsaolateral prefrontal cortex
Functions in. Executive decision making

BA 47—found in the frontal lobe on the orbital surface
Functions in the processing of syntax

BA 52—found in the temporal lobe in the lateral sulcus
Functions in auditory processing

REFERENCES

Abraham, C.R., Selkoe, D.J., and Potter, H. 1988. Immunohistochemical identification of the serine protease inhibitor alpha 1 antichymyotrypsin in the brain amyloid deposits in Alzheimer's disease. Cell 52:487-501

Adams R.D., and Victor M., 1989. Principles of Neurology, 4th ed. New York: McGraw-Hill.

Albin R.L., A.B. Young and J.B. Penny. The Functional Anatomy of the Basal Ganglia Origin. Trends Neurosci. 1989 12: pp. 366-379.

Allen G.I. and Uskahara N., 1974. Cereberocerebellar communication systems. Physiol. Rev. 54:957-1006.

Armstrong C.M., 1981. Sodium channels and gating currents. Physiol. Rev. 61:644-683.

Ashby P., and M. Wiens. Reciprocal Inhibition Following Lesions of the Spinal Cord in Man. J. Physiol., 1989. 414:pp. 145-157.

Barrett J.N., 1975. Motorneuron dendrites: Role in synaptic integration. Efd. Proc. 34:1398-1407.

Beal, M.F., and Martin, J.B. 1986 Neuropeptides in neurological disease. Ann. Neurol. 20:547-565.erapy, 2nd ed. New York: Plenum Press.

Benton,A.,Tranel,D.Visuoperceptual,viseospatial,andviseoconstructional disorders. Clinical neuropsychology, 3rd ed. New York: Oxford University Press 1993:165.

Bellugi U, Poizner H, Klima ES,. Brain organization for language: clues from sign aphasia. Hum. Neurobiol. 1983:2:155.

Bertroud H.R., and W.L. Neuhuber. Functional and Chemical Anatomy of the Afferent Vagal System. Autonomic Neurosci., 200. 85(1-3):pp. 1-17.

Bickford, R.G., Mulder, D.W., Dodge, H.W., Jr., Svien, H.J., and Rome, H.P. 1958 Changes in memory function produced by electrical stimulation of the temporal lobe in man. Res. Publ. Assoc. Nerv. Ment. Dis. 36:227-243.

Blodel, J.R., Bracha, V., Kelly, T.M., Wu, Jin-Zi. 1991. Substrates for motor learning. Does the Cerebellum do it all? Ann NY Acad. Sci. 627:305-318.

Brown P., Pathophysiology of Spasticity. *J. Neurol. Neurosurg. Psychiatry.* 1994. 57: pp. 475-495.

Brodal P., The Central Nervous System. 1998. Oxford University Press: New York. 1998.

Brodal A., 1981. Neurological Anatomy In Relation to Clinical Medicine, 3rd ed. New York: Oxford University Press.

Carpenter M.B., and SutinJ., 1983. Human Neuroanatomy, 8th ed. Baltimore. Williams & Wilkins.

Catteral W. A., 1988 Structure and function of voltage sensitive ion channels. Science 242:50-61.

Clark, R.G., Anatomy of the mammalian cord. *In handbook of the spinal cord.* Vol. 2. R.A. Davidoff. New York, Marcel Dekker, Inc. pp 1-46. 1984.

Cohen, D.H., 1982. Central processing time for a conditioned response in a vertebrate model system. Representations of Involved Neural Functions. New York; Plenum press, pp. 517-534.

Cordo P.J., Nashner L.M., 1982. Properties of postural adjustments associated with rapid arm movements J. Neurophysiol. 47:287-302.

Cote, L.J., and Kremenzner, L.T. 1983. Biochemical changes in normal aging in human brains. The Dementias. Advances in Neurlogy, Vol 38. New York; Raven Press, pp. 19-30

Cowen W.M., 1979. The development of the brain. Sci. Am. 241(3):112-133.

Crystal, H., Dickson, D., Fuld P., Massur, D., 1988 Clinopathologic studies in dementia: Nondemented subjects with pathologically confirmed Alzheimer's disease. Neurology 38:1682-87.

Davies, P. 1986. The genetics of Alzheimer's disease: A review and discussion of the implications. Neurobiolo. Aging7: 459-466.

Damasio AR. Aphasia. N Engl J Med 1992:326-531.

Damasio AR., Tranel D., Verbs and nouns are retrived with differently distributed neural systems. PNAS 1993:90:4957

Damasio AR., Anderson SW., The frontal lobes Clinical Neuropsychology 3rd ed. New York: Oxford University Press 1993:409.

Damasio, AR., Van Hoesen GW., Emotional disturbances associated with focal lesions of the limbic frontal lobe. Neurophyschology of human emotion. New York: Guilford Press, 1983:85.

Dastur D.K., Lane M.H., Hansen D.B., Kety S.S., Effects of aging on cerebral circulation and metabolism in man. Human aging: A Biological and Behavioral Study. Public Health Service Publ. No. 986 Waashington, DC: US Government Printing Office, pp. 57-76. Trends Neurosci. 1990. 13: pp. 281-285.

Domjan M., and Burkhaed B., 1982 The Principles of Learning and Behavior. Monterey, California: Brookes/Cole.

Evans BA., Stevens JC., Dyck PJ., Lumbosacral plexus neuropathy. Neurology 1981: 31:1327-1331.

Edelman R.R., Magnetic resonance imaging of the nervous system. Discus. Neurosci. 7:11-63.

Fields H.L., 1987. Pain. New York: McGraw Hill.

Giardino L., M. Zanni, M. Fernandez, A. Battaglia, O. Pigntaro, and L. Calza. Plasticity of GABAa System During Aging: Focus on Vestibular Compensation and Possible Pharmacologic Innervention. *Braain Res.* 2002. 929

Graf P., Mandler G., and Haden P.E., 1982. Simulating amnesic symptoms in normal subjects. Science 218:1243-1244.

Goetz, C.G., and E.J. Pappert. Textbook of Clinical Neurology. 1999 W.B. Saunders Co. Philadelphia.

Goldman J.E., and Yen S.E., Cytoskeletal protein abnormalities in neurodegenerative disease. Ann Neurol. 19:209-223.(1986)

Goodale M.A., and A.D. Miller. Separate Pathways for Perception and Action *Trends Neurosci.* 1992. 15(1):pp. 20-25.

Gottlieb G. (editor) Studies on the Development of Behavior and the Nervous System. Academic Press, New York. (Volume 1)1973.

Haines D.E., Neuroanatomy, An Atlas of Structures, Sections and Systems. 3rd ed. Urban & Schwarzneberg. Baltimore—Munic, pp. 252 (1991).

Hardy A.G., and Rossier A.B., Spinal Cord Injuries. Georg Thieme Publishers, Stuttgart. (1975).

Hayflick L., The Cell biology of human aging. Sci. Am. 242(1):58-65.

Heimer L., 1983. The Human Brain and Spinal Cord: Functional Neuroanatomy and dissection Guide. New York. Springer.

Hilgard E.R., and Bower G.H., 1975. Theories of Learning. 4th ed. Englewood Cliffs, N.J.: Prentis-Hall.

Hodgkin A.L., 1964. The Conduction of the nervous Impulse. Springfield Ill.: Thomas ch. 4.

Hokefelt T., Fuxe K., Pernow B., (editors) Coexistance of Neuronal Messengers: A New Principle in Chemical Transmission, Progress in Brain Research. Vol. 68, Elsevier Publishing Company, Amsterdam.

Hudspeth A., 1989. How the ear's works work. Nature 341:397-404.

Hullinger M., The Mammalian Muscle Spindle and Its Central Control. Rev. Physiol. Biochem. Pharmacol., 1984. 101:pp 1-110.

Humphery D.R., W.S. Corrie. Properties of Prymidal Tract Neuron System within functionally Defined Subregion of Primate Motor Cortex. J. Neurophys., 1978:41:pp. 216-243.

Iuarto S. 1967. Submicroscopic Structure of the Inner Ear. Oxford University Press.

Jacobson M., Developmental Neurobiology, 2nd ed. Plenium Press, New York. (1978)

Karam D, Biochemical Principles for the Medical Student. Indiana: Trafford Press 2012, 188-193.

Klatzky R.L,. 1980. Human memory: Structures and processes, 2nd ed. San Francisco: Freeman.

Kuypers H.G., 1973The anatomical organization of the descending pathways and their contribution to motor control especially in primates. New Developments in Electromyography and Clinical Neurophysiology, Vol 3. Basel: Karger, pp. 38-68.

Krnjevic M., Neurotransmitters in the Cerebral Cortex. Cerebral Cortex. Plenum Press, New York, 2:39-61.

Linas R., and Jahnsen H., 1982. Electrophysiology of mammalian thalamic neurons in vitro. Nature 297:406-430.

Lorente De. The Structure of the Cerebral Cortex. Physiology of the Nervous System. Ed 3. Oxford University Press, New York, pp. 288-330. 1949.

Lwzak MD., Neuropsychological assessment, 2nd ed. New York: Oxford University Press 1983.

Ludwin S.K., Norman M.G., Congential malformations of the nervous system. In Textbook of Neuropathology R.L. Davis and D.M. Robertson (editors) Williams & Wilkins, Baltimore pp. 176-242.

Marr D., 1969. A theory of the cerebellar cortex. J Physiol. (Lond.) 202:437-470.

Martin J.H., Neuroanatomy: Text and Atlas. New York: Elsevier.

Medvedev Zh. Repetetion of molecular-genetic information as a possible factor in evolutionary changes in life span. Exp. Gerontol. 7:227-238.

Merton P.A., Merton H.B., 1980. Stimulation of the cerebral cortex in human subjects. Nature 285:227.

McCrea D.A. Spinal Circuitry of Sensorimotor Control of Locomotion. *J. Physiol.* 2001. 533(1) pp. 11-18.

McGaugh J.L., 1989. Involvement of hormonal and neuromodulatory systems in the regulation of memory storage. Annu. Rev. Neurosci. 12:255-287.

McGeer P.L Eccles J.C., McGeer E.G. Molecular Neurobiology of the Mammalian Brain 2nd ed. Plenum Press, New York, pp. 744. A. Davis, 1985:125

Moore K.L., The Developing Human: Clinically Oriented Embryology. 4th ed. W.B. Sanders Co., Philadelphia.

Mountcastle V.B., Effects of Spinal Transection. In Medical Physiology, Vol 1, 13th ed. V.B. Mountcastle (editor) C.V. Mosby Co., St. Louis, MO, pp662-667. (1974)

Nashold B.S>, Ostdahl R.H., 1979. Dorsal root entry zone lesions for pain relief. J Neurosurg. 51:59-69.

Osborn A.G., Introduction to Cerebral Angiography. Harper & Row, Publishers, Hagerstown, Maryland pp. 436.

Pavlov I.P., 1927 Conditional reflexes: An investigation of the Physiologic Activity of the Cerebral Cortex. London: Oxford University Press.

Pearson R.C., Esiri M.M., Hiorns R.W., Wilcock G.K., Anatomical Correlates of the distribution of the pathological changes in the neocortex in Alzheimer's disease and related dementia. Neurosci. Comment. 1(2):84-92.

Penfield W. and Rasmussen T., 1950. The cerebral cortex of man: A clinical Study of Localization of Function. New York. Macmilliam.

Perry E.K., Perry R.H., Blessed G., Necropsy evidence of central cholinergic deficits in senile dementia. Lancet 1:189. 1977.

PhelpsM.E., Mazziotta J.c., and Huang S.C.,. 1982 Study of cerebral function with positron computed tomography. J Cereb. Blood Flow Metab. 2:113-162.

Porter R. and R. Lemon. *Cortical Function and Voluntary Movement.* 1993. Clarendon Press: Oxford.

Preston J.B, and Whitlock D.G., 1961. Intracellular potentials recorded from motorneurons following precentral gyrus stimulation in primates. J. Neurophysiol. 24:91-100.

Rexed B., Some aspects of the cytoarchitectonics and synaptology of the spinal cord. Progress in Brain Research, Vol. 11. Organization of the Spinal Cord J.C. Eccles and J.P. Schade(editors) Elseviever Publishing Company, Amsterdam. Pp. 58-92.

Ruda M.A., Bennet G.J., and Dubner R., 1986. Neurochemistry and neural circuitry in the dorsal horn. Prog. Brain Res. 66:19-268.

Schneider J.S., S.G. Diamond, and C.H. Markham. *Parkinson's Disease: Sensory and Motor Problems in Hands and Feet.* Neurology, 1987, 37.

Scoville WB., Milner B. Loss of recent memory after bilateral hippocampal lesions. J Neurol Neurosurg Psychiatry 1957;20:11. The neural basis of basic associative learning of discreet behavioral responses. Trends Neurosci. 11:152-155.

Selkoe D.J., The molecular pathology of Alzheimer's disease. Neuron 6:487-498. 1991.

Selkoe D.J., Amyloid Protein and Alzheimer's Disease. Sci. AM. 265(5):68-78. 1991

Sokolov L. 1984. Modeling metabolic processes in the brain in vivo. Ann. Neurol. [Suppl] 15:S1-S11.

Shepard G.M., 1988. Neurobiology, 2nd ed. New York: Oxford University Press.

Sherrington C. 1947. The Integrative Action of the nervous System, 2nd ed. New Haven: Yale University Press.

Sherrington C. 1898. Decerebrate rigidity and reflex coordination of movements. J. Physiol. (London) 22:319-332.

Somjen G., 1972. Sensory Coding in the Mammalian Nervous System. New York: Appleton—Century—Croft.

Siegel G., Agranoff R., Alberts W., Molinoff (editors) Basic Neurochemistry 4th ed. Raven Press, New York, pp. 984 (1989).

Stephen R.B., and Stilwell D.L., Arteries and Veins of the Human Brain. (1969) Charles C. Thomas, Springfield, Illinois

Stryer L., Bourne H.R., G-Proteins: A family of signal transducers. Ann. Rev Cell Biol., 2:391-413.

Schnitzlein H.N., and Murtagh F.R., Imaging Anatomy og the Head and Spine. Urban & Schwarzenberg, Baltimore—Munich. (1985).

Schibel A.B., The organization of the spinal cord. *In Handbook of the Spinal Cord*, Vol 2 R.A. Davidoff (editor). Marcel Dekker, Inc., New York, pp. 47-78.

Thatch W.T., 1978. Correlation of neural discharge with pattern and force of muscular activity, joint position, and direction of intended next movement in motor cortex and cerebellum. J Neurophysiol. 41:654-676.

Topka H., L.G. Cohen, R.A., Hallet. Reorganization of Corticospinal pathways Following Spinal Cord Injury. Neurology, 1991. 41(8): pp. 1276-1283.

Tranel D., Daaasio AR., The learning of affective valance does not require structures in the hippocampal system. Journal of Cognitive Neuroscience 1993;5:79.

Tulving E., and Schacter D.L., Priming and human memory systems. Science 247:301-306. 1990. Press, 198etinotopic organization of areas 18 and 19 in the cat J. Comp. Neurol., 185:657-678.

Vitek, J.L., V. Chockan, J.Y. Ahang, Y. Kaneoke, M. Evatt, M.R. DeLong, S. Triche, K. Mewes, T. shimoto, and R.A. Bakay. Neuronal Activity in the Basal Ganglia in Patients with Generalized Dystonia and Hemiballismus. Ann. Neurol., 1999. 46(1):pp 22-35.

Wall P.D., and Melzack R. (eds) 1989. Textbook of Pain, 2nd ed. Edinburg: Churchill Livingstone.

Weikrantz L., 1986 Blindsight: A case study and implications. Oxford. Clarendon Press.

Werner G., and Whitsel B.L., 1973. Functional Organization of the somatosensory cortex. In A. Iggo(ed) Handbook of Sensory Physiology, Vol 2: Somatosensory System. New York: Springer, pp. 621-700.

Wu, W.J, S.H. Sha, J.D., Schacht. Recent Advances in Understanding Aminoglycoside Ototoxicity and its Prevention. *Audil. Neurotol.* 2002. 7(171-174).

Yeung AC., Moore MR., Goldberg A. Pathogenesis of acute porphyria. Q J Med 1987; 163:377-392.

Yool A.J., and Schwartz T.L., 1991. Alteration of ionic selectivity of a K+ channel by mutation of the H5 region. Nature349:700-704.

Yoshida M., A. Rabin, and A. Anderson. Monosynaptic Inhibition of Pallidial Neurons by Axon Collaterals of Caudatonigral Fibers. *Exp. Brain Res.* 1972. 15:pp. 33-347.

Young RR., Shahani BT. Asterixis: One type of negative myoclonus. Adv. Neurol 1986; 137-156.